TYPE 1 DIABETES
MENTAL HEALTH
WORKBOOK

A Practical Resource for Providing Behavioral and
Mental Health Support to Young People with
Type 1 Diabetes, and Their Families

Kimberly A. Driscoll, PhD

Marisa E. Hilliard, PhD

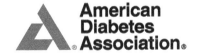

American
Diabetes
Association®

Director, Book Operations, Victor Van Beuren; *Associate Director/Managing Editor, Books*, John Clark; *Director, Book Marketing*, Annette Reape; *Editorial Services*, Absolute Services; *Printer*, Lightning Source.

Printed in the United States of America

1 3 5 7 9 10 8 6 4 2

The suggestions and information contained in this publication are generally consistent with the *Standards of Medical Care in Diabetes* and other policies of the American Diabetes Association, but they do not represent the policy or position of the Association or any of its boards or committees. Reasonable steps have been taken to ensure the accuracy of the information presented. However, the American Diabetes Association cannot ensure the safety or efficacy of any product or service described in this publication. Individuals are advised to consult a physician or other appropriate health care professional before undertaking any diet or exercise program or taking any medication referred to in this publication. Professionals must use and apply their own professional judgment, experience, and training and should not rely solely on the information contained in this publication before prescribing any diet, exercise, or medication. The American Diabetes Association—its officers, directors, employees, volunteers, and members—assumes no responsibility or liability for personal or other injury, loss, or damage that may result from the suggestions or information in this publication.

♾ The paper in this publication meets the requirements of the ANSI Standard Z39.48-1992 (permanence of paper).

American Diabetes Association titles may be purchased for business or promotional use or for special sales. To purchase more than 50 copies of this book at a discount, or for custom editions of this book with your logo, contact the American Diabetes Association at the bulk book sales address below, at booksales@diabetes.org, or by calling 703-299-2046.

American Diabetes Association
Bulk Book Sales
PO Box 7023
Merrifield, Virginia 22116-7023

American Diabetes Association
2451 Crystal Drive, Suite 900
Arlington, VA 22202

DOI: 10.2337/9781580408189

Library of Congress Control Number: 2023938559

Contents

Preface ix

Definitions xi

Chapter 1 Overview of T1D 1

    Diabetes Technology 4

    Orientation to Mental Health Care in T1D 4

    Developmental Considerations of T1D Self-Management. 6

Chapter 2 Language and Communication about T1D 9

    Supportive Communication 9

    Shaming and Blaming 10

Chapter 2 Worksheets. 13

    Using "I Messages" 15

    My New Name for T1D. 17

    Family Glucose Communication Plan 19

Chapter 3 Challenges Associated with a New T1D Diagnosis. 21

Chapter 3 Worksheets. 23

    My T1D. 25

    Letter for Teens 27

    Write a Letter to Your Future Self. 29

    Letter for Caregivers. 31

    Diaversary Party Checklist 33

Chapter 4 Approaches to Addressing T1D Self-Management Challenges 35

    Creating Routines to Support T1D Management. 37

T1D-Specific Family Conflict 41

T1D-Specific Interventions 43

Chapter 4 Worksheets 45

What Goes in Your Kit? 47

My T1D Team 49

Setting SMART T1D Management Goals 51

Problem-Solving Steps for T1D Management Challenges 53

The IDEAL Way to Problem Solve T1D Management Challenges 55

Problem-Solving and SMART Goal-Setting for T1D
Management Challenges 57

Problem-Solving T1D Challenges Using Pros and Cons 59

Child's Morning Routine 61

Child's Morning Routine Items 63

Child's Bedtime Routine 65

Child's Bedtime Routine Items 67

Adolescent Routine 69

Adolescent Morning Routine 71

Adolescent Evening Routine 73

Reward Chart 75

Chapter 5 Emotions Associated with T1D 77

Common Emotional Responses in Youth 77

Strategies to Navigate Emotional Responses to T1D 78

Chapter 5 Worksheets 81

What Are Your Emotional Triggers 83

Chapter 6 Mood Concerns and T1D 85

Depression 85

Diabetes Distress 85

Treating Depression and Diabetes Distress 86

Suicide Risk 87

Chapter 6 Worksheets 91

Child Safety Planning and Coping Skills 93

Teen/Young Adult Safety Planning and Coping Skills 95

Think-Feel-Do 97

Chapter 7 T1D-Related Worries and Anxiety 105

T1D-Specific Social Anxiety 105

Fear of Hypoglycemia 105

Needle Anxiety and Blood Phobia in Individuals with T1D 111

Treating T1D-Related Worries and Anxiety 112

Chapter 7 Worksheets 115

CBT for Fear of Hypoglycemia 117

Challenging Unhelpful Thoughts 119

Alternative Thoughts 121

Math Exercise 123

Cognition Cartoon 125

Fear Ladder 127

Fear Ladder Items 129

Practicing Exposures 137

Fear Thermometer 139

Chapter 8 Additional Considerations 141

Pain 141

Sleep 142

Supporting Siblings of Youth with T1D 143

Chapter 8 Worksheets. 145

Getting a Good Night's Sleep with T1D 147

Resources 149

References 153

Contributors

Katherine Gallagher, PhD
Baylor College of Medicine and Texas Children's Hospital
Houston, TX

Jessica Kichler, PhD
University of Windsor
Windsor, Ontario
Canada

Maureen Monaghan, PhD
Children's National Hospital and George Washington University School of Medicine
Washington, DC

Diana Naranjo, PhD
Stanford University School of Medicine
Stanford, CA

Holly O'Donnell, PhD
Barbara Davis Center for Diabetes
University of Colorado
Aurora, CO

Sarah Westen, PhD
University of Florida
Gainesville, FL

Preface

Living with a complex chronic health condition like type 1 diabetes (T1D) is complicated, expensive, and burdensome. Most people live long, happy, healthy, satisfying lives with T1D, yet there is a large body of evidence (from research, clinical practice, and personal experience) that mental health concerns and behavioral challenges are common and interfere with self-management, quality of life, and health. Although the American Diabetes Association and other professional diabetes organizations recommend integrated mental and behavioral health support as part of routine diabetes care, there are not enough professionals in these fields who have knowledge of the complex interplays between diabetes and psychosocial factors to meet the needs of the large and growing population of people with T1D, and their families.

To address this shortage, one of us (Marisa) was a member of the steering committee to develop and implement a structured educational program through the American Diabetes Association for licensed mental health professionals to learn about diabetes. The American Diabetes Association's Diabetes Education 101 for the Behavioral Health Provider Program, which provides mental health professionals with the knowledge they need to deliver assessment and intervention to individuals with T1D, as well as members of their families and extended social support networks, is now available as a video-on-demand program. This online program offers continuing education credits (https://professional.diabetes.org/meetings/mental-health-provider-diabetes-education-video-demand-program). While serving as speakers for several in-person workshops, we recognized the need for a workbook to supplement this program, which mental health clinicians and therapists could use to guide their care of young people with T1D. We enlisted a team of pediatric psychologists with expertise in T1D to contribute to the content of this resource, and together we created a brief, practical workbook that summarizes the key clinical, mental, and behavioral health concerns of pediatric T1D, spanning early childhood through early adulthood, and provides techniques and tools for implementation in practice. The prevalence of type 2 diabetes (T2D) in pediatrics has been increasing, and although this book does not specifically focus on the concerns of patients with T2D, many of the concepts apply. We are pleased to provide this workbook for mental health providers that contains content specific to T1D.

This workbook is structured into eight chapters: 1) Overview of T1D; 2) Language and communication about T1D; 3) Challenges associated with a new T1D diagnosis; 4) Approaches to addressing T1D self-management challenges; 5) Emotions associated with T1D; 6) Mood concerns and T1D; 7) T1D-related worries and anxiety; and 8) Additional considerations. Each chapter includes a brief introduction to the chapter topic based on scientific evidence and our clinical and research experiences along with those of our coauthors. We are all licensed clinical psychologists with research and clinical expertise in T1D. Embedded throughout the introductory text are tables, figures, and content examples. At the end of each section within a chapter are customizable worksheets to be used as part of a therapy session. Worksheets make sessions with child and adolescent patients more engaging and encourage creativity and communication. Downloadable PDF versions of these worksheets are available free of charge on the American Diabetes Association's website, ShopDiabetes.org.

We also provide a resources section that includes information on organizations, books, and websites that we find to be helpful for us and the individuals and families with whom we work. Throughout the workbook, we incorporate content related to family dynamics, child and adolescent development, and diversity, cultural, and systems factors that may influence the topics and your provision of mental and behavioral healthcare. We include the best available research in the field, which we acknowledge is limited by underrepresentation of youth and families from racially and ethnically minoritized groups or from low socioeconomic backgrounds. We recognize that access to high-quality healthcare for diabetes is a privilege that not all people with T1D have, especially with the high costs of insulin, inequitable coverage of diabetes management devices, and bias throughout the healthcare system. Access to a mental health professional who has received education about T1D is even less common, especially because insurance coverage of mental healthcare is highly variable across states and often inadequate. Our hope is that changes in the healthcare system, policies, and society reduce systemic barriers to the most effective medical and mental healthcare for all people, including youth with T1D, as well as their families.

Kimberly A. Driscoll, PhD
Director of Behavioral Science Research,
University of Florida Diabetes Institute, Gainesville, FL;
Department of Clinical and Health Psychology,
University of Florida, Gainesville, FL

Marisa E. Hilliard, PhD
Baylor College of Medicine and Texas Children's Hospital,
Department of Pediatrics, Division of Psychology, Houston, TX

.

Definitions

Acute complications: Short-term effects of out of range blood glucose, including hyperglycemia, hypoglycemia, diabetic ketoacidosis, seizure, and coma.

Automated insulin delivery system: Also known as "artificial pancreas," "closed-loop," or "hybrid closed-loop." These systems include a connected insulin pump and continuous glucose monitor with a software algorithm that adjusts insulin delivery based on current and predicted glucose.

Basal and bolus insulin: Basal insulin is long-acting or intermediate insulin administered once a day to regulate glucose throughout the day. Bolus insulin is short- or rapid-acting insulin administered at mealtimes to regulate glucose fluctuations with food intake or when glucose is too high. A basal–bolus insulin regimen is designed to mimic the functioning of a pancreas without T1D.

Blood glucose meter: Device used to measure current blood glucose using a droplet of blood from a fingerstick.

Continuous glucose monitor: Device worn on the body to measure interstitial glucose every 5 minutes. A sensor is positioned on the skin that includes a cannula (i.e., a tiny plastic tube penetrating the skin) that measures glucose, which is visible on a separate handheld display or smartphone app.

Diabetes distress: A common emotional response to the everyday burdens, challenges, and stressors related to living with and managing T1D. There are some similarities to depressive symptoms, but diabetes distress is related specifically to diabetes.

Diabetic ketoacidosis: Serious acute complication of hyperglycemia in which the body begins to burn fat and muscle for energy. Blood acids called ketones are produced and coma or death may occur.

Fear of hypoglycemia: Concern about the potential risk of low blood glucose level. Moderate amounts of fear may be adaptive and may lead to appropriate self-management behaviors; extremely high fear may interfere with functioning.

Glycemic variability: Increases and decreases in blood glucose outside the recommended range (usually 70–180 mg/dL).

Hemoglobin A1c (A1C): Blood test indicating average glucose during the past 2–3 months and a common marker of overall diabetes-related health. The American Diabetes Association A1C target for most people is <7.0%.

Hyperglycemia: Blood glucose above the target range (usually >180 mg/dL).

Hypoglycemia and severe hypoglycemia: Blood glucose below the target range (usually <70 mg/dL). Severe hypoglycemia is an urgent safety situation when the person with diabetes requires assistance from another person, often <54 mg/dL.

Insulin pump: Device worn on the body that administers insulin through a cannula that penetrates the skin. Some models communicate directly with glucose data from a continuous glucose monitor, see "Automated insulin delivery system."

Long-term complications: Health consequences of diabetes across time, including problems with the heart, eyes, nerves, reproductive organs, and other health systems.

Time in range: Percent of time one's glucose is in the target range (usually 70–180 mg/dL) throughout a specified period, calculated from continuous glucose monitor readings.

Chapter 1
Overview of T1D

Type 1 diabetes (T1D) requires constant monitoring and management of blood glucose. Specific tasks conducted multiple times a day by individuals with T1D (or parents of youth with T1D) include checking blood glucose via fingerstick or continuous glucose monitor, calculating and administering insulin doses via injections or insulin pumps, possibly taking additional medications to regulate blood glucose, paying attention to dietary intake, carbohydrate counting and administering the appropriate amount of insulin needed with every meal and snack, and making decisions about engaging in physical activities.[1]

Incomplete cognitive development prevents young people with T1D from always recognizing healthful choices or behaving in a way that promotes health and minimizes short- and long-term complications.[2] Indeed, as children transition into adolescence, engagement in T1D self-management tasks often decreases and A1C increases.[3,4] This pattern occurs despite significant advancements in diabetes technology, in part due to generally low uptake and use and inequities for people with low socioeconomic status and from racially and ethnically marginalized groups, particularly with the continuous glucose monitor.[5] Given the many behavioral and psychosocial factors (e.g., cognitive development, family interactions, motivation, behavioral reinforcement) that are related to patterns of deterioration in T1D self-management and worsening glycemic outcomes during the adolescent years, mental health professionals are well-suited to help young people with T1D improve self-management behaviors as well as physical and psychological health outcomes.[6]

Ideally, a person with T1D will have glucose in the target range of 70–180 mg/dL at least 50%–60% of the time, with almost no time with glucose <70 mg/dL (i.e., low blood glucose or hypoglycemia), minimal time with glucose between 181 and 399 mg/dL (i.e., high blood glucose or hyperglycemia), and no time with glucose >400 mg/dL.[7] However, hypoglycemic and hyperglycemic episodes inevitably occur and are often accompanied by unpleasant physical symptoms including dizziness, rapid heartbeat, and confusion (with hypoglycemia) or fatigue, nausea, increased thirst and urination, and fruity-smelling breath (with hyperglycemia). Severe or sustained hypoglycemia or hyperglycemia have potentially dangerous outcomes including seizure, coma, or death.

To prevent such serious and deleterious outcomes, the American Diabetes Association recommends an A1C of <7% [8]; however, targets may vary based on individual circumstances and as recommended by a medical provider. Most children, adolescents, and young adults do not have an A1C within this target[3] and there are greater disparities in glycemic outcomes for Black and Hispanic youth.[9] A variety of factors such as food intake, stress, hormone fluctuations, and illness affect blood glucose. Careful execution of T1D-related tasks reduces the risk of acute medical events, including severe hyperglycemia or hypoglycemia, diabetic ketoacidosis, seizure, coma, and death, and of long-term health complications, including retinopathy/blindness, neuropathy (e.g., erectile dysfunction, amputation), nephropathy/kidney failure, cardiovascular complications (e.g., high blood pressure, heart disease, stroke, heart attack), and premature death.

The American Diabetes Association's *Standards of Care in Diabetes* include medical treatment guidelines and nutrition recommendations for youth with T1D.[8,10] Individuals with T1D must administer insulin exogenously using multiple daily injections via syringes, insulin pens or insulin pumps, with insulin being short-acting, rapid-acting, or long-acting. Insulin is administered to lower elevated blood glucose, ideally to the target glucose range. Attempts to lower persistently elevated blood glucose can result in administering too much insulin through the pump or "stacking insulin" when using multiple daily injections. This is colloquially referred to as a "rage bolus,"[11] referring to the urge, usually based in fear or frustration, to repeatedly give more insulin to try to decrease a persistent high blood glucose. Continuing to administer an insulin dose before the insulin has time to work can eventually lead to a dangerously low blood glucose event. Addressing the low blood glucose requires eating food high in carbohydrate or ingesting glucose tablets or gels, which can then result in another blood glucose spike (colloquially known as a "rebound high"), resulting in a frustrating and exhausting rollercoaster effect. Mental health professionals can assist with preventing these blood glucose extremes and emotionally driven behavioral responses, especially when the primary referral for treatment is for improving self-management behaviors.

Striking a balance among blood glucose, carbohydrate intake, insulin delivery, and physical activity is important for T1D self-management. Given the complexity of dietary management in T1D, behavioral support for food and eating is a critical part of self-management. Foods with high carbohydrate, such as starches, fruit, and milk, raise blood glucose the most. Vegetables have low carbohydrate; meats and cheeses contain little or no carbohydrate. Proteins and fats can also affect blood glucose, although not as rapidly. One of the most challenging aspects of managing T1D is meal planning, especially when eating at a restaurant or if food delivery is delayed. A meal plan should be created with input from the child's endocrinologist and an experienced registered dietitian and should include insulin delivery.

The American Diabetes Association emphasizes that registered dietitians/registered dietitian nutritionists should be the primary providers of medical nutrition therapy for individuals with T1D and that medical providers should refer all people with T1D to these specialists for an individualized nutrition plan.[10] Food choices involve multifaceted considerations (e.g., personal preferences, developmental stage, cultural traditions) and, for some families, may be controversial, with important health consequences, so it is important for the child to follow the medical team's advice.[12] Mental health professionals should not give medical advice about what to eat, but, in partnership with the diabetes care team (especially registered dietitians), mental health professionals can work with youth and their families to address behavioral and psychosocial challenges and facilitate implementation of the medical nutrition recommendations (e.g., managing child behavior at mealtimes).

Attending routine healthcare visits with T1D specialists (e.g., endocrinologists, diabetologists, diabetes educators, registered dietitians) and other medical professionals (e.g., dentistry, ophthalmology) is necessary to promote optimal health outcomes for people with T1D. Considering the American Diabetes Association recommendations for quarterly assessment of A1C, which typically occurs during a T1D care visit,[1] estimating 15–45 minutes per visit, youth with T1D are likely to receive 1–3 hours of direct medical care from a diabetes healthcare professional per year. Healthcare access barriers (e.g., distance from medical center, inadequate insurance coverage) may reduce the amount of T1D medical care young people receive.

Even so, the majority of T1D care is accomplished through self-management and conducted by the person with T1D in the context of everyday life. Data from the U.S. National Survey of Children with Special Health Care Needs showed that ~33% of families of children with T1D reported spending 11 or more hours per week completing T1D management tasks.[13] This may be an underestimate: the experience of parents of young children with T1D is described as "constant vigilance."[14]

In addition to attending clinic appointments, T1D self-management involves maintaining an adequate amount of diabetes management supplies, including insulin, blood glucose monitoring supplies (e.g., glucose meter, testing strips, alcohol wipes, lancing device, continuous glucose monitor and associated supplies, ketone testing supplies), insulin delivery supplies (e.g., syringes, insulin pens, insulin pumps and associated supplies), treatments for low glucose (e.g., glucose tablets, emergency glucagon kit, snacks), and other medications. Not only are many supplies necessary, but they come from different manufacturers, have different expiration dates, and many require prescriptions and insurance authorizations. Their costs are high, making it difficult for many families to afford the life-sustaining medical supplies T1D treatment requires.[15–17] It is well-known that many individuals with T1D ration their supplies for financial reasons,[17] and many people engage in "underground" sharing of supplies, prescriptions, and devices to reduce the high costs,[15] which is a significant source of stress.[18,19] When working with a child and family with relatively low engagement in T1D self-management, the mental health professional must determine whether the family cannot afford glucose test strips, insulin, sensors, and other supplies.

Supplies Needed to Manage T1D		
Glucose Monitoring	Meter Strips Lancing Device Alcohol wipes	Continuous glucose monitors Sensor Transmitter/phone

Carbohydrates	Fast-acting sugar
	  Juice
	  Candy
	  Cake gel
	  Glucose tabs
		Snacks
		Apps to count tabs

Insulin	Vials
	Syringes
	Pens
	Alcohol wipes
		Insulin pump
		  Infusion sets
		  Cartridges

Other	Glucagon Ketone strips Medical bracelet/necklace Other medications	

Diabetes Technology

Diabetes devices include blood glucose meters, continuous glucose monitors, insulin pumps (also known as continuous subcutaneous insulin infusion), insulin pens, sensor-augmented insulin pumps, and closed-loop (or hybrid closed-loop) insulin pumps. These technologies allow for greater awareness of glucose patterns, easier insulin calculations and dosing, increased flexibility around meals, less attention to T1D in social situations, and better sleep.[20-24] However, there are also clinical challenges related to diabetes devices use, especially for youth. Barriers to starting devices and maintaining use include physical discomfort when wearing devices, self-consciousness about device visibility, frustration with device errors and malfunctions, interference with activities, and high costs.[24,25] There are also significant disparities in device access and use in racially and ethnically minoritized groups and groups with low socioeconomic status,[26,27] which may help explain disparities in glycemic outcomes across these groups.[28] Systemic barriers (e.g., healthcare coverage), and implicit bias among providers leading to sharing information about devices differentially, likely contribute to disparities.[29,30]

Youth and their parents may have different expectations for how the devices will affect their lives, perspectives on the value of using a diabetes device, or preferences about which devices to use or how to use them. If parents and youth differ in terms of acceptance about wearing a device, a useful strategy may be to complete an activity to help the family brainstorm short-term versus long-term costs and benefits of wearing a device from each person's perspective, which may help to frame preferences, priorities, and expectations for each device.

Many diabetes devices have options for remote monitoring, in which wearers make data accessible to others, such as parents, through Bluetooth connections (known colloquially as 'sharing'). This gives parents and other support persons real-time access to glucose and trends (i.e., increasing, decreasing, stable), which can be useful when children and adolescents are away from parents (e.g., at daycare/school or sleepovers, with babysitters, during sports). However, constant access to diabetes data can also increase worry about glycemic extremes, contribute to family conflict about T1D, or encourage parents to 'micromanage' T1D remotely. It is important to consider the reasons for using remote monitoring and what is developmentally appropriate for each child at different stages of development (e.g., the age-appropriate level of parental oversight for an adolescent or young adult who is transitioning to college or already independently managing T1D self-care). Mental health professionals can help families establish boundaries around sharing glucose data by negotiating agreements about access and methods of communication.

Orientation to Mental Health Care in T1D

Mental health professionals, including psychologists, psychiatrists, social workers, counselors, and other providers with training in psychology or behavioral health, are key players in multidisciplinary care for youth with T1D and their family members.[6,31] The daily demands of living with and managing T1D can take an emotional toll on young people and their parents and loved ones.[32,33]

Many psychological, behavioral, cognitive, developmental, family, socioeconomic, and environmental factors affect whether and how much young people and their families engage in the complex health behaviors required of the T1D management regimen.[34] Family relationships play a critical role in T1D management; completely independent self-management is not a realistic expectation for most youth.[35,36] The training and expertise of mental health professionals make them ideally suited to assist families by using empirically supported behavioral interventions to support high quality of life and encourage high engagement in T1D self-management behaviors; thus, mental health professional support is a vital part of promoting optimal T1D-related health.[6,37] The American Diabetes Association's *Standards of Care in Diabetes* (updated annually)[8] and *Psychosocial Care for People With Diabetes* position statement,[38] as well as guidelines from international diabetes organizations,[39] call for involvement of mental health professionals in routine psychosocial monitoring and care.

Mental health professionals caring for youth with T1D may work in a variety of settings. In large academic medical centers with diabetes care services, multidisciplinary care teams may include social workers and at least one psychologist. In these settings, mental health professionals may provide fully integrated care within the medical clinic setting, mental health care in the same physical location as the medical care, or coordinated care in which they provide mental health services by referral in a separate physical location. Mental health professionals may treat people with T1D outside of medical systems,[40] such as those who work in community mental health centers, agencies, or private/group practices who receive referrals from healthcare providers or other sources. Arrangements vary widely; 72% of pediatric diabetes care providers report "easy access" to mental health services, whereas only slightly more than 50% have mental health professionals as part of the multidisciplinary team.[41]

Mental health professionals who care for people with T1D provide a variety of services, including screening, assessment, and treatment of mental health conditions and behavioral health concerns related to living with T1D, family conflict related to T1D and its management, challenges related to T1D self-management behaviors, and preparation for transition to adult healthcare for young people and their families.[6,42] Treatments include brief interventions integrated into medical clinics, traditional outpatient treatment (e.g., individual, group, family), brief treatment during inpatient hospitalizations, and professional consultation with healthcare providers.[6,43]

One of the critical considerations for mental health professionals working with youth and families is understanding shifts in T1D-related behavioral and psychosocial experiences across different developmental stages.[35] Young people mature at different rates, and the decision to add responsibilities for T1D self-management should be personalized based on the youth's and family's interest, T1D knowledge, self-management skills/abilities, and comfort. The following tables outline considerations for youth engagement and parents' roles in T1D self-management tasks at different developmental stages. Within the chapters in this workbook, we offer developmental perspectives on these topics.

Mental health professionals are also well-situated to address a range of social determinants of health related to diabetes management and outcomes.[44] In addition to addressing mental health concerns, mental health professionals help young people with T1D and their families cope with stressors related to socioeconomic inequities and systemic discrimination, overcome barriers to heath behaviors attributable to environmental limitations or neighborhood disadvantage, and seek support from social systems and community resources. Mental health professionals also often partner with care coordinators, social workers, and other members of diabetes care teams to address other social determinants of health, such as food insecurity, economic stability, and navigating complex healthcare systems.

Developmental Considerations of T1D Self-Management Tasks

Children (≤8 Years of Age)

Because they have limited skills across several domains, children mostly rely on parents for T1D management and to detect and treat glucose fluctuations. Primary mental health targets typically include parental distress and child behavior management.[45]

Developmental Characteristics of Children	Effects on T1D-Related Tasks	Parental Roles
Period of rapid growth (physical, cognitive, social)	Children are learning to communicate about feelings, including feeling "low"	Monitoring glucose and behavior to detect changes in insulin needs
Developing autonomy; may say "no"	May resist some diabetes management tasks; children do not have self-regulation skills to perform T1D management tasks without adult oversight	Implementing behavior management strategies and maintaining consistent routines; helping child get involved in minor T1D management tasks
Unpredictable eating habits and activity	Can make insulin dosing difficult to determine	Monitoring food intake and physical activity; managing mealtime behavior
May spend time with other caregivers, such as child care providers, grandparents, babysitters, and friends	Children are unable to perform T1D management tasks independently; parents may not know whether other caregivers understand enough about T1D to manage it effectively	Educating other caregivers about diabetes management tasks and establishing a communication plan

Pre/early Adolescents (9–12 Years of Age)

Developing abilities for completing health behaviors (including T1D self-management tasks) requires close adult supervision and assistance. Primary mental health targets typically include self-consciousness about T1D, learning T1D self-management tasks, and establishing effective communication patterns about T1D with parents.[46]

Developmental Characteristics of Pre/Early Adolescents	Effects on T1D-Related Tasks	Parental Roles
More social, may spend more time away from parents, may be self-conscious about T1D	May complete glucose checks or basic self-management tasks when apart from parents; still needs adult oversight	Supporting social relationships; helping young people learn basic self-management skills to conduct in social settings; arranging alternate adult oversight
Increasing responsibility and self-management skills	Can learn carbohydrate counting, with adult confirmation; may be able to recognize and treat lows	Continuing to share responsibilities; encouraging involvement in activities (e.g., sports, school activities) with plan for T1D management and adult supervision
Understands consequences	Can communicate about barriers to T1D self-management when away from parents; may have ideas or need help to resolve them	Encouraging and modeling problem-solving skills for T1D challenges

Adolescents (13–17 Years of Age)

Self-management skills are increasing but executive functioning skills are not fully developed in this stage; therefore, adolescents need adult support and oversight. Increasing mood concerns and distress (which may involve disordered eating behaviors, body image concerns, and self-consciousness) and social interference with self-management are common, as is increased family conflict about T1D self-management. Major mental health-care targets typically include mood, family relationships, self-management skills, and preparation for transitioning to autonomous self-care. Most intervention research in this area demonstrates limited long-term effects.[47]

Developmental Characteristics of Adolescents	Effects on T1D-Related Tasks	Parental Roles
Increasing autonomy and self-management skills	Can begin completing the majority of self-management tasks	Ongoing adult support and monitoring of T1D management is necessary
Developing identity, increasing self-consciousness in social settings	Can make decisions about diabetes self-management (e.g., technology)	Encouraging family collaboration/partnership for T1D management; emphasizing social support for the adolescent
May engage in risky behaviors; executive functioning skills still in development	Can think of solutions for problems with input from parents	Enforcing limits and consequences
Increasing demands from school, peer relationships, and extracurricular activities	Increasing understanding of importance of prioritizing T1D care for future health	Avoiding nagging; establishing communication plan that is agreeable to parents and the adolescent
Mood swings	T1D challenges are normal	Checking in regularly about health and mood

Young/Emerging Adults (18–25 Years of Age)

Young adults have many competing demands and simultaneous changes across many domains (including their T1D), may be changing healthcare providers, and may exhibit mood concerns, distress, or disordered eating behaviors. Major mental health care targets typically include managing many stressors, talking to new people about diabetes, navigating relationships, and support for transitioning to autonomous self-care.[47]

Developmental Characteristics of Young/Emerging Adults	Effects on T1D-Related Tasks	Parental Roles
Establishing identity after high school; many competing priorities; may move away from home	Telling new people about T1D; advocating for T1D needs in school/work settings	Supporting transition to adulthood; assisting with information and skills as needed
May become more independent from parents	Transitioning to adult medical care	Supporting transition from pediatric to adult T1D care
Solidifying executive functioning and problem-solving skills and skills for self-management	Responsible for daily self-management tasks, integrating T1D into new lifestyle	Continuing to provide emotional support and assistance when needed

Chapter 2
Language and Communication About T1D

It is critical for professionals working with people with T1D and their family members to use the most current, nonjudgmental, professional language to communicate with respect and understanding. The Association of Diabetes Care & Education Specialists and American Diabetes Association developed language use guidelines for diabetes care and education consisting of five anchoring principles.[48] Whereas people with T1D may use their own preferred terminology to talk about themselves or their experiences with T1D (e.g., "diabetic," "bad blood sugars"), we recommend professionals adhere to these guidelines consistently.

Use Language that Fosters Collaboration

- Neutral, Nonjudgmental & Based on Facts
- Free from Stigma
- Strengths Based, Respectful, Inclusive, and Imparts Hope
- Person Centered

Language choices can be a useful intervention target when working with children with T1D and their parents. Words like "noncompliant" can sound accusatory or judgmental when used by medical providers. Similarly, adolescents may perceive parents' use of language as judgmental or disapproving, which can lead to conflict and difficulty with collaborative teamwork when managing T1D.[49]

People with T1D have many characteristics besides having diabetes, thus, it is important to use inclusive, person-centered language in reference to race, ethnicity, gender identity, sexual orientation, ability, socioeconomic status, and the intersections among them.[50]

Supportive Communication

The way we communicate with each other has a direct effect on how we feel about ourselves and others. Therefore, it is important to establish ground rules about communication and to do so early when a child is diagnosed with T1D, particularly teaching the use of "I messages," in which the person speaking asserts his or her own thoughts, feelings, beliefs, or values (see the "Using I messages" worksheet). A mental health professional can

Say this...not that!

Say this	...not that!
Person with type 1 diabetes	Type 1 Diabetic
High/low blood glucose/ A1c	Bad/good blood glucose, A1C
Completing some, not all, T1D tasks	Noncompliant
Chronic hyperglycemia	Uncontrolled type 1 diabetes

assist family members to learn to communicate effectively about T1D. For example, parents can be encouraged to talk with their young children about whether they feel "different" living with T1D, or about any worries or frustrations they have about completing T1D self-management tasks (e.g., checking blood glucose, carbohydrate counting, giving insulin, wearing devices). For adolescents, teaching skills to improve their communication may be necessary to reduce perceptions that the parent is 'nagging' or being critical.

For example, adolescents may not want to be asked about T1D as soon as they come home from school, but may prefer to communicate about T1D-related updates via text messages or to sit with a parent and talk about T1D updates before dinner. To prevent and manage conflict, family members should start T1D-related conversations when calm, give everyone a

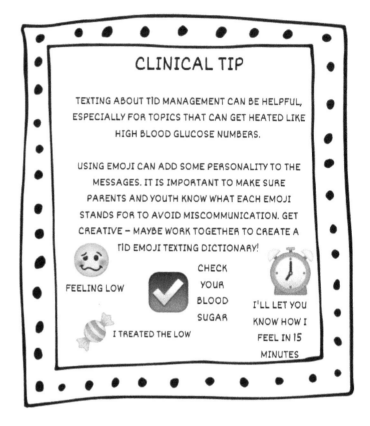

chance to think about their ideas before talking, and take breaks to return to calmness when a conversation leads to conflict. Agreeing on preferred words, framing of questions, and times to talk about T1D can help families avoid misspeaking and triggering conflict. These foundations of positive communication, with coaching from a mental health professional, have the potential to improve T1D management interactions and ultimately improve health.

Use of text messaging (with emojis) for communication about T1D may be helpful for youth and parents who find that their discussions about blood glucose numbers and self-management behaviors escalate into arguments. Similarly, many parents find their children are most open and forthcoming about T1D when they are driving in the car; sitting side by side rather than having direct, sustained eye contact may help reduce tension or pressure that could arise in these conversations.

Shaming and Blaming

Parents may need to be taught to avoid using shaming or blaming language when discussing T1D care (i.e., "What did you eat to get numbers this high?" "He's always lying about giving his insulin." "She just doesn't care about T1D at all and I'm tired of it.") Young people with T1D may internalize messages of shame and blame and use this language as well. Whereas this kind of language usually reflects the speaker's fears and frustrations about how difficult it can be to live with and manage T1D, it shifts the blame for the difficulty of T1D from the disease to the person with T1D and communicates that the person with T1D is failing. When parents (or professionals) use shaming and blaming language, children are likely to feel ashamed, embarrassed, or misunderstood, and may attempt to hide information about T1D management to avoid continuing to feel that way (e.g., by omitting information or being dishonest about blood glucose numbers, giving insulin, or food that was eaten). It is important to acknowledge and normalize emotions that shaming and blaming language often mask failure, disappointment, frustration, anger, and fear. When mental health professionals help youth and parents express these feelings, the conversation can shift from one that is accusatory to one that is supportive, and negative emotion can be

Clinical Tip

It is not unusual for parents to adopt "Should Statements" like

My child SHOULD remember T1D supplies.

My child SHOULD be able to take care of all T1D tasks.

My child SHOULD stop eating pizza so her blood glucose doesn't increase.

Help parents to manage expectations and consider that their child may not be ready for full T1D responsibility.

redirected toward the true source of the feelings: T1D. Similarly, it is important to recognize that children's behaviors in reaction to shame and blame (e.g., hiding T1D information) are logical and adaptive for them, and often developmentally appropriate. As a mental health provider, your work to help families find more effective ways to communicate about T1D that avoid shaming and blaming will likely improve not only communication, but also engagement in T1D self-management behaviors.

One strategy that some people with T1D and their family members use in an attempt to separate the child from T1D (and thus avoid feeling blamed and shamed) is to give T1D a name. For example, one child we counseled named her T1D "Acacia." Whenever her blood glucose was higher or lower than she wanted, she and her parents would say, "Acacia is not being helpful today," or "Acacia is being a brat!" rather than blaming the child for doing something wrong. Mental health professionals are in an ideal position to suggest creative, age-appropriate activities like this to help people use language in a way that will minimize negative feelings related to T1D (see the "My new name for T1D" worksheet).

Chapter 2 Worksheets

Use an I Message to:
1. Tell what is happening.
2. State how you feel.
3. Explain why you feel that way.

I Messages are a good way to share how you're feeling without placing blame or shame. Try using these statements to increase positive communication and understand others' perspectives!

When _____, I feel _____ because _____.

When _____, I feel _____ because _____.

When _____, I feel _____ because _____.

When I have to go to the nurse's office before lunch, I feel worried and stressed because I miss the end of my Spanish class and can't write down the homework.

When I get constant reminders to check my blood glucose, I feel frustrated because I don't get the get the chance to show how I can check my blood glucose on my own.

MY NEW NAME FOR T1D

write down some different names and then pick one!

HELLO
my name is

HELLO
my name is

HELLO
my name is

HELLO
my name is

HELLO
my name is

why did you pick this name?

_____

_____

Family Glucose Communication Plan

What do we need?

1. Meter or visual display of glucose values
2. Calm attitude

What else do you need?

When do we do it?

Find a time to meet that works for your family at least 3x per week. Before dinner? After soccer? Set a day and time and stick to it!

1.
2.
3.

What do we do?

1. Have your numbers ready (e.g., meter, device report, device app).
2. Look for patterns.
3. Talk about what you see.
4. What things can you change?

Remember BG values are *just* numbers, not grades. Stay calm and look for the positive!

Tips!

1. Write the meetings on a calendar or in your phone.
2. Set communication rules for meetings.
3. Meet at the same time and in the same place.
4. Eliminate distractions.
5. Use problem-solving techniques as needed.

Based on Monaghan, M., Clary, L. Mehta, P., et al. (2015). Checking In: A pilot of a physician-delivered intervention to increase parent-adolescent communication about blood glucose monitoring. *Clinical Pediatrics, 54*(4), 1346-1353.

Chapter 3
Challenges Associated with a
New T1D Diagnosis

A new T1D diagnosis may provoke profound grief in young children, parents, and other family members, leading to feelings of shock, denial, anxiety, sadness, guilt, anger, and frustration.[51] Grief may focus on loss of a formerly healthy status, loss of control, and loss of freedom in daily activities. Often there is disbelief that T1D is permanent, worry about acute and long-term health complications, and guilt that either the person with T1D or their parents caused T1D through genetics or actions (e.g., food choices). The newly diagnosed individual becomes a person with T1D; parents have a new focus on caring for a child with a lifelong, possibly life-threatening condition. In addition, a new T1D diagnosis necessitates learning and integrating many new health-behavior routines into daily life. An exercise that may help children identify or express feelings about a new diagnosis is to draw their T1D (see the "My T1D" worksheet) or write a letter to T1D (see the "Letter to T1D" worksheet for adolescents). This same exercise may also be helpful for caregivers (see the corresponding caregiver worksheets).

Mental health professionals can offer anticipatory guidance that there may not be a discrete end point to this grief. Symptoms of grief may ebb and flow across time. Grief may resurface when developmental milestones are met and as adolescents transition to young adulthood. Grief may also recur when there are challenges or changes in T1D management such as a T1D-related medical event or hospitalization or learning new technology. Triggers related to the initial T1D diagnosis may include the anniversary of the diagnosis (sometimes referred to as "Diaversary") or learning about other people's T1D challenges or the death of a person with T1D. Chronic unresolved grief has the potential to lead to diabetes distress or depressive symptoms. Guiding young children and parents to consider these possibilities around the time of the initial T1D diagnosis may help them anticipate and prepare for possible resurgence of grief. Some people benefit from using positive psychology-based approaches, such as recognizing or "celebrating" annual "Diaversaries" as a chance to reflect on how far they have come since diagnosis (see the "Diaversary party checklist" worksheet).

Children who experience very high stress at diagnosis are most likely to experience poorer quality of life and have ongoing emotional challenges,[52] especially during the first year after diagnosis.[53] Clinical intervention strategies that target improving stress management include 1) developing a new routine, 2) relaxation and calming skills, 3) use of flexible and creative problem-solving techniques, and 4) positive reframing strategies.[54] In addition to general stress management interventions, resilience-building interventions can be powerful tools for adjusting to a new diagnosis and for those who struggle with overcoming obstacles to T1D management.[55] Resilience intervention techniques focus on enhancing and promoting individuals' positive attributes and strengths. For example, resilience-building mental health interventions increase one's sense of self-efficacy (the person is capable of handling obstacles associated with managing T1D) and self-mastery (the person has the skills to complete T1D self-management tasks and emotionally process any setbacks), promote optimism, and help the individual recognize how new skills help one overcome challenges.[55]

Adjustment to the losses associated with a T1D diagnosis does not necessarily represent a resolution of grief or stressors. Rather, adjustment reflects an acceptance about living with all of the emotions associated with T1D by experiencing them rather than avoiding them. People develop acceptance of the challenges of living with T1D at a different pace and in different ways. Indicators of increasing T1D acceptance may include a child explaining T1D basics to classmates or friends, an adolescent feeling comfortable wearing diabetes devices that are visible to others, or a young adult taking ownership of T1D-related tasks when transitioning to college.

Chapter 3 Worksheets

Let's draw T1D. What does T1D look like? What does T1D feel like? What does T1D tell you? T1D might look like a cartoon, a color, or a person. Your drawing of T1D can be anything!

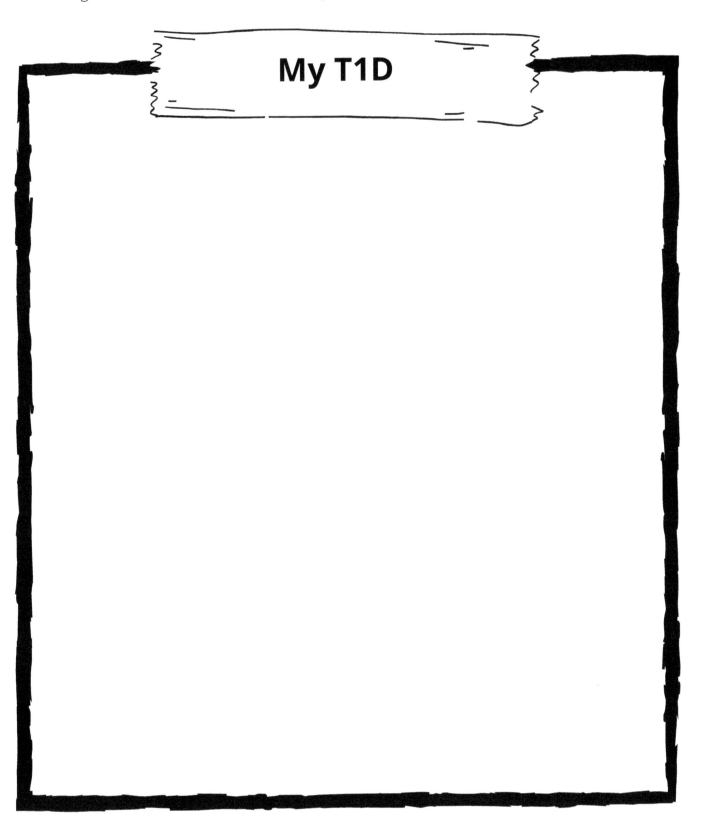

My T1D

For Teens: Writing down our feelings can help us feel better. To help "take the emotion out of T1D," write a letter to your T1D. What do you want to tell your T1D? What thoughts do you have about your T1D? What feelings do you have about your T1D?

Dear T1D,

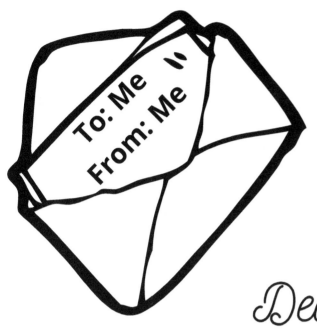

Write a Letter to Your Future Self

Instructions: Write a letter to your future self. Write whatever you want– nobody will see it. Seal it in an envelope, put it somewhere safe, and read it in 6 to 12 months.

Dear Future Self,

Values: What things are important to me? What do I hope I am doing with T1D in 6 to 12 months?

Actions: What T1D goals do I want to work on between now and when I read this letter again?

Barriers: What thoughts and feelings may get in the way of reaching these goals?

Strategies: What can I do to reach my T1D goals?

Adapted from *The Diabetes Lifestyle Book: Facing Your Fears and Making Changes for a Long and Healthy Life.* By Gregg, Callaghan, & Hayes (2007)

For Caregivers: Writing down our feelings can help us feel better. To help "take the emotion out of T1D," write a letter to your child's T1D. What do you want to tell your child's T1D? What thoughts do you have about your child's T1D? What feelings do you have about your child's T1D?

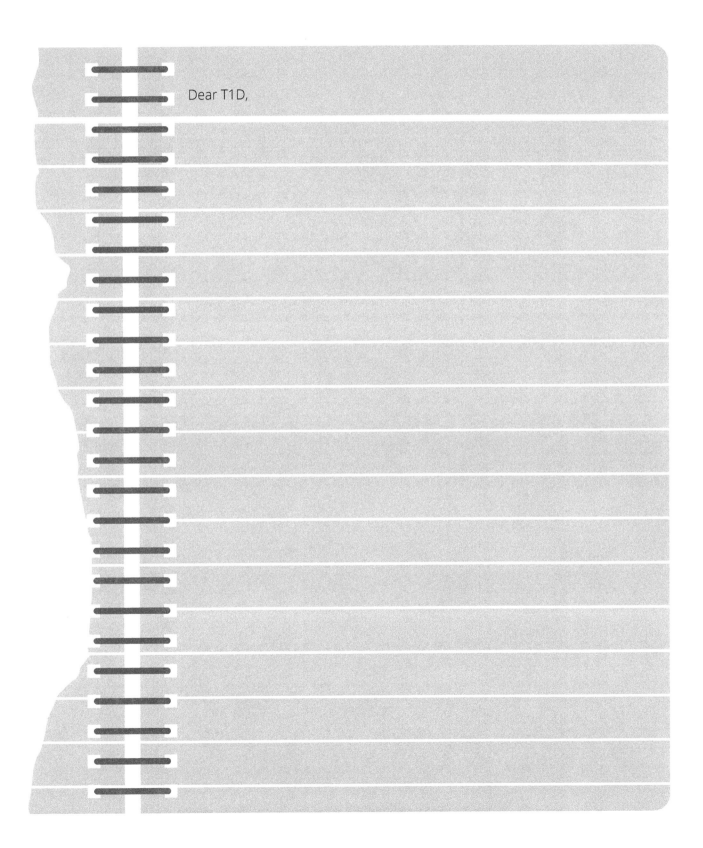

Dear T1D,

DIAVERSARY PARTY CHECKLIST

Set date

Decide on the guest list

Decide on theme

Decide on place

Send invitations

Paper plates, utensils, napkins

Balloons

Food

Cake

Insulin!

NOTES

Chapter 4
Approaches to Addressing T1D Self-Management Challenges

T1D management is too complex and demanding to be a 'do-it-yourself' project. Youth from early childhood through young adulthood have improved medical and psychosocial outcomes when parents are consistently involved in T1D care in a positive and developmentally appropriate way.[35,36]

Parental involvement in the child's T1D care includes providing tangible, emotional, and logistical support related to living with and managing T1D. The needs for and specific roles of parents will change as the child grows and gains more self-management skills. Identifying members of the family's T1D team is essential at all developmental stages of the child's life (see the "T1D team" worksheet).

Throughout early childhood and into adolescence, parents evolve from being care providers who complete most of the daily T1D management tasks to managers who perform some T1D-related tasks (e.g., scheduling medical appointments, sick day management) directly while overseeing other T1D-related tasks (e.g., reviewing carbohydrate counting, double-checking insulin dosing) to coaches who provide support for the child's completion of T1D-related tasks.[36] To ensure that T1D management tasks are completed consistently across time, progression toward independence should happen in tandem with the child learning how to complete daily management tasks and gradually taking the lead on completing those tasks.

Parent and Child Involvement in T1D Tasks	
Young Childhood	Allow child to choose • a new location for insulin pump set change • between a few snack choices
School Age	Parents should • Be present and observe completion of tasks • Provide instruction and guidance • Step in and give hands-on assistance when needed • Provide frequent, positive reinforcement even if child cannot complete a task on their own • Be flexible and plan for events like sleepovers and parties
Late Childhood – Early Adolescence	Parents should • Monitor T1D management when possible – through physical presence and observation, and/or checking in via conversation, text-messaging, or T1D apps • Offer support and help with solving T1D management problems • Provide frequent praise and support for successfully completing tasks – NOT the numbers!

Parents of very young children with T1D take primary responsibility for all T1D care tasks,[45] but young children can be involved in their care. For example, young children can assist by selecting which finger to use for a blood glucose check or lining up supplies for a device site change. Because so much responsibility for constant T1D management falls to parents during early childhood, it is important that parents receive support from other family members, friends, healthcare professionals, and other adults. It is common for parents' needs to be overlooked because their child is the focus of the medical provider's attention; however, some may need their own mental health provider to address unresolved grief, symptoms of anxiety or depression, or stress.

As children reach school age, they start to learn the basics of T1D self-management and may have increasing involvement in carrying out some daily T1D self-management tasks, such as using their lancet for a glucose check, alerting parents or caregivers if they feel symptoms of hypoglycemia, and preparing supplies for site changes for diabetes devices. It is important for parents to remain as involved in T1D management routines as possible even as children become more able to complete tasks. School-aged children likely have the manual dexterity to perform some tasks (e.g., checking blood glucose, drawing up insulin dose) but are still advancing their cognitive skills related to more complicated tasks related to T1D, such as calculating insulin doses and carbohydrate counting for meals. In late childhood and early adolescence, children may begin to become more actively involved in daily T1D self-management tasks, including administering insulin injections/boluses with parental oversight, carbohydrate counting with parent confirmation, and telling others about T1D.

By late adolescence and early young adulthood, many youth take primary responsibility for daily T1D care tasks. Some may also become responsible for tasks that occur less frequently, such as sick-day management, ordering T1D supplies, scheduling T1D medical appointments, and managing challenges related to health insurance.[56] The process of transferring responsibility for T1D care tasks from primarily the parent to primarily the adolescent or young adult should be gradual, occurring throughout many years and ideally with consistent parental monitoring and support.[57] At no point should T1D management be solely the responsibility of the person with T1D.

Sometimes younger children are given too much responsibility for T1D management too quickly or do not receive enough supervision, monitoring, or support for their T1D management responsibility. A premature transition of responsibility is associated with negative health outcomes including elevated A1C.[57-59] Decisions about responsibility should not be driven simply by the child's age; considerations should include the young person's maturity level, T1D duration, demonstrated mastery of self-management tasks, psychosocial functioning, cognitive capabilities, family or cultural expectations for developing independence, specific environments (e.g., school, camp, sports), and other factors that might interfere with or facilitate T1D management. It is critical to remember that developmental stages are generalizations and each child and family may have different needs and skills that should guide the expectations for what the child is able to do for T1D self-management. For example, people who are diagnosed later in childhood or adolescence may not complete as many tasks independently as younger children who have had T1D for several years.

Whereas T1D management responsibility shifts gradually from parents to the child, the process is not always unidirectional or linear. It is normal for there to be periods of time when children are less able to prioritize T1D management or could use more hands-on assistance from family members. Mental health professionals can assist with setting reasonable expectations for how families share T1D care responsibilities. More family teamwork may be needed temporarily when other demands are high (e.g., during final examinations) or when children experience periods of diabetes distress or burnout related to the unrelenting demands of daily T1D management.[32] At times, parents may need to provide more supervision, support, or direct care to give their child a break from T1D, with parents checking blood glucose, calculating insulin doses, carbohydrate counting, administering insulin injections/boluses, or handling diabetes device site changes. Ensuring that there is an active backup support team providing daily oversight, monitoring, and emotional support for diabetes care responsibilities is essential.

It is also critical to recognize that there may be specific facilitators of and barriers to parental involvement for children from different racial, ethnic, or socioeconomic backgrounds, such as unpredictable or inflexible work schedules, acculturation, generational status/immigration recency, traditional family roles, cultural expectations for youth autonomy, and support through community groups or churches.[60,61] Tailored assessment of each family's particular circumstances and perspectives about parental involvement in T1D management at different ages is important for mental health professionals to coach families in providing optimal levels and types of oversight for the child's diabetes self-management.

Friends and romantic partners also play an important role in T1D management, particularly for adolescents and young adults. Interacting with other people with T1D through activities such as T1D camps is associated with reduced diabetes distress and increased engagement in T1D self-management behaviors.[62] Children and parents from racially and ethnically minoritized backgrounds report fewer social support systems for T1D and there are significant racial and ethnic and socioeconomic disparities,[63] especially among children who attend camp,[64,65] which may limit opportunities for accessing support from peers with T1D. Negative peer interactions characterized by T1D conflict are associated with more negative diabetes outcomes.[62] Young adults with T1D may seek support from romantic partners and friends; supportive peer and partner relationships are associated with better adjustment.[66] Mental health professionals can assist with the identification of friends and romantic partners to provide T1D support. Given the fluctuating nature of relationships during these stages, enlisting the support of long-term friends and partners in stable relationships who have demonstrated interest in being a T1D supporter may be most effective.

Creating Routines to Support T1D Management

Establishing routines around T1D self-management tasks facilitates behavioral patterns that make T1D management easier. Routines incorporate structure, timing, planning, and support from others.[67] For T1D, this includes repeated series of self-management behaviors that occur on a consistent or regular schedule, including checking blood glucose and giving insulin (multiple times per day), reviewing blood glucose patterns (weekly), reviewing diabetes supplies for expiration dates and quantity (monthly), and attending routine medical visits (quarterly). In contrast to routines, habits are acquired modes of behavior that occur almost automatically and without thinking in response to a cue.[68] Some routines may become habits; for example, a parent of a young child with T1D may automatically look at a food label or start carbohydrate counting at every meal. Mental health professionals can help people with T1D establish routines and build habits that help integrate T1D self-management into their activities in a way that works for them. Completing self-management tasks consistently—at the same time, in the same order, or in response to specific prompts—is a central strategy to integrate T1D self-management tasks into daily life. Conversely, having less-established routines or experiencing unexpected disruptions to routines can introduce T1D self-management challenges.

T1D self-management routines and overall family organization are associated with better T1D outcomes[69–71] and may facilitate ongoing family involvement in a child's T1D management across racial and ethnic groups.[72] As children grow and schedules change, routines may need to be adapted or modified to meet the family's needs. For younger children, routines also reduce behavioral challenges related to T1D care.[73] Families may notice more T1D self-management challenges during periods of developmental transitions and when routines are changing, such as when young children start a new school or when adolescents are becoming more independent and responsible for their T1D care. For young adults, changes to school and work schedules, inconsistent sleep and activity patterns, changing social and romantic relationships, and other disruptions interfere with T1D self-management routines.[74] Times when there are

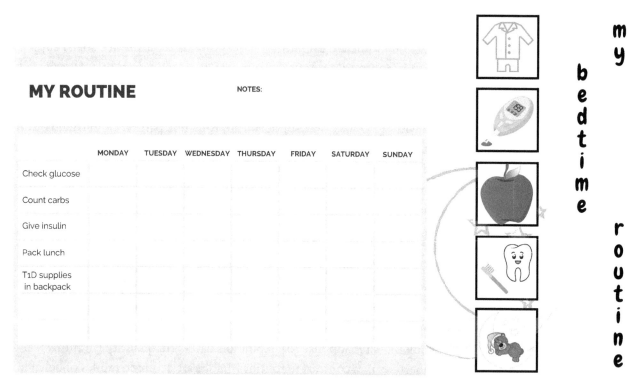

Example of adolescent routine worksheet   Example of child's bedtime routine worksheet

changes in T1D treatments (e.g., starting a new device, using a different insulin type) may introduce challenges for established T1D management routines at all ages.

Mental health professionals promote successful health routines by assessing individual and family functioning, recent and anticipated stressors or schedule changes, strengths and areas in need of improvement, motivations, and organizational strategies.

Beginning this process with an assessment of current T1D routines offers insight into both established routines and routines that may need improvement. Using open-ended questions to ask families about current routines, what is working well, and where challenges may occur, as well as standardized questionnaires, can help identify which T1D-specific tasks may be targets for intervention.[70] This information can guide tailored, structured approaches to help the child and family select activities or reminders that meet their needs and daily schedules. A variety of worksheets to create routines are provided at the end of this section for children (cards that can be cut out and put in order of needed completion) and adolescents (list format).

Intervention approaches to promote successful routines include the following:[67]

Reeducation involves creating, establishing, and sustaining a new routine. This is particularly challenging when there are no prior successful routines in place or when the family struggles with organization. When a person is newly diagnosed, all T1D management tasks will fall in this category of routine development.

Remediation occurs when a new behavior is integrated into an existing routine. For a young child with T1D who is starting a new diabetes device, this may include creating a routine to change a pump insertion site at the same time that the child is already changing a continuous glucose monitoring site.

Redefinition of a routine is needed when a routine is disrupted, possibly by a change in schedule or developmental transition, and needs to be redefined to meet the new circumstances. For example, an adolescent with T1D may start a weekend evening job, necessitating administering insulin and eating dinner 30 minutes earlier than usual to ensure on-time arrival.

Realignment occurs when different family members or environments have conflicting views on a routine or about its importance, such as when a child lives in two households with each parent taking different approaches to T1D care or when parental involvement varies. In these cases, all caregivers should work together to negotiate an agreement framed as being in the child's best health interest, but mental health professionals may need to help with this process.

To establish or modify health behavior routines, it is important to identify specific and individual steps needed to accomplish the routine. Breaking the routine into individual parts clarifies what is needed. For example, young children may benefit from an illustrated checklist or schedule describing each step of a T1D care task (see "My T1D Kit" figure and associated worksheet at the end of this chapter).

It also helps to pair a routine with a trigger or an already established activity that matches the child's everyday activities and developmental stage (i.e., the Premack principle). Examples include placing a blood glucose meter on the nightstand to help the child remember to check blood glucose upon awakening and before bed, or placing it near a toothbrush to pair blood glucose checking with dental hygiene routines.

Pairing T1D care tasks with enjoyable, predictable activities, such as feeding a pet,[76] can improve T1D self-management for some children.[75] As a new T1D self-management behavior routine is established, it is important to track progress, celebrate successes, identify challenges, and adjust the routine as needed.

My T1D Kit

- ☐ blood glucose meter
- ☐ insulin
- ☐ pens and needles for injections
- ☐ fast acting sugar
- ☐ snacks
- ☐ extra supplies for technology (pumps, continuous glucose monitor)

Triggers for checking blood glucose ...

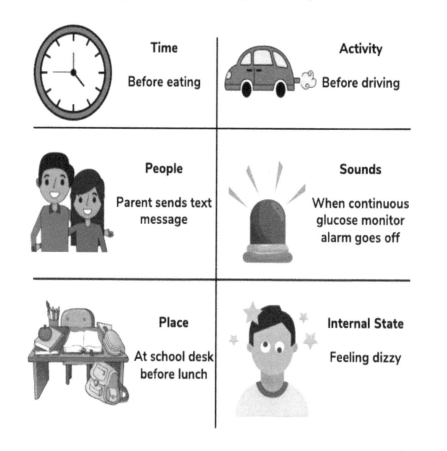

Time
Before eating

Activity
Before driving

People
Parent sends text message

Sounds
When continuous glucose monitor alarm goes off

Place
At school desk before lunch

Internal State
Feeling dizzy

T1D-Specific Family Conflict

For young children with T1D, working together with caregivers to manage T1D brings its own challenges. Arguments or disagreements about T1D-related tasks are a common consequence of the demands and worries associated with T1D. In fact, T1D-specific family conflict is one of the most common reasons that youth with T1D are referred for mental health services.[77] Persistent or intense T1D-specific conflict is associated with multiple negative health outcomes[78] and is one of the strongest predictors of high A1C among adolescents.[78,79]

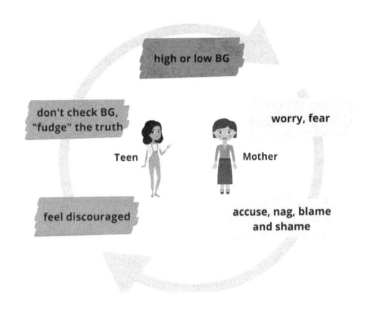

Family conflict generally arises out of a desire to help with T1D care and often escalates during adolescence, the developmental period marked by a desire for increased independence and focus on peers, which has significant implications for daily T1D self-management.[58]

Conflict also arises when there is a mismatch between a child's developmental abilities in relation to T1D care and caregiver expectations (i.e., when parents expect children to take on more responsibility for T1D self-management than they are able to).[80] Family members often try to be helpful but end up unintentionally exacerbating a problem. In addition, parents may use ineffective approaches, such as strictness, overprotection, and harshness,[36] which increase the potential for conflict.

Parents worry about their child and their child's health and want to do everything they can to keep their child healthy and to prevent diabetes complications. However, when children perceive their parents' worries and fears as negative, judgmental, intrusive, or punitive,[81] they are likely to withdraw and withhold information (to avoid unpleasant interactions with the parent). The withholding contributes to continued negative interactions, making it difficult for parents to be involved collaboratively in T1D management tasks. Conflict may persist into young adulthood, when increasing independence for T1D self-management and general health occurs, but prioritizing T1D care in the context of other responsibilities may be difficult.[82]

Mental health professionals may observe T1D-specific family conflict during an initial evaluation or as T1D challenges are discussed. For example, an adolescent may not make eye contact or engage in conversation about T1D care and a parent may use blaming or shaming language to discuss the child's T1D care (see the *Language and communication about T1D* chapter). Often caregivers present for a mental health consultation because their child is "lying" about glucose numbers, "sneaking food," or not communicating about T1D care when spending time with peers or away from the family home. Children may report that a parent is constantly nagging them about T1D management. All family members may express feelings of frustration, anger, or hopelessness about how to improve family interactions surrounding T1D care.

Mental health professionals can address these issues using many of the same tools that are used to address family conflict about challenges not related to T1D.

Reframing behaviors to use more positive language and reduce negative emotions about T1D are important first steps. Youth may not check blood glucose or disclose numbers that are out of range because they are worried, disappointed, or anticipate a negative reaction from a parent or healthcare provider. Rather than saying that the child is being dishonest about glucose numbers, reframing is needed to acknowledge that eating without telling a parent may occur to avoid a negative reaction or being told "no." The mental health provider's goal is to help the family use positive, collaborative problem-solving skills to recognize this pattern and develop new ways to address the child's needs (e.g., desire to eat and need for insulin) and respond to out-of-range glucose numbers.

Changing behaviors related to T1D management can be difficult but is a central role of mental health professionals in the care of youth with T1D and their families. Reinforcement is used to increase or maintain behavior and is recommended for promoting behavior change.

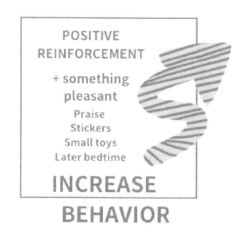

Positive reinforcement means rewarding a desired behavior to encourage engagement in that behavior again. Given the important consequences of suboptimal T1D management, it is common for parents and healthcare professionals to focus much attention on missed T1D self-management tasks and blood glucose values that are outside of the target range. Mental health providers can help parents refocus their attention on what their child with T1D does well for T1D management and reinforce positive T1D-related behaviors instead. For example, parents should use specific verbal and nonverbal praise, such as saying "I'm so proud of you for giving your shot!" while giving the child a high-five. Parents of a teenager or young adult can send a text message, such as "👍 I saw you changed your pump site! You rock 🩸." This is a good opportunity to use the decided-upon communication plan or emojis to indicate appreciation of completing T1D self-management tasks (see the *Language and communication about T1D* chapter).

When establishing specific behavioral goals, offering tangible rewards may increase a desired behavior for many youth. For example, a parent may develop a token system for the child to earn a small gift or privilege (e.g., screen time) for completing T1D-related tasks such as checking blood glucose on an agreed-upon schedule. It is essential that the reward is valuable to the recipient so that it motivates completion of the desired behavior. Each family will have a different level of comfort with, or resources, to be able to provide tangible rewards, so it is important to talk with parents about this before discussing this in a session with the child present.

Some parents and caregivers may think of positive reinforcement and providing rewards as bribery, so it is important to talk with parents about these terms: bribery involves using illegal methods to coerce someone to engage in a negative behavior, whereas positive reinforcement involves using agreed-upon methods to encourage someone to work towards a reward by engaging in a positive behavior. Using the analogy of adults working for a paycheck may help parents think differently about "bribing" their children and reframe rewards as positive reinforcement.

Punishment is used to decrease behavior, but it is typically less effective than positive reinforcement for promoting health behavior change. Punishment typically involves removing something meaningful to decrease a behavior. For example, if a teenager talks back to a parent every time the parent asks if the teenager has their T1D supplies, the teenager may have their cell phone taken away in an effort to decrease talking back. Punishment should never be used in response to an out-of-range blood glucose number or A1C. It is important that behavior change techniques be used to support self-management behaviors, not glucose readings or A1C.

T1D-Specific Interventions

There are two evidence-based, behavioral family-focused intervention protocols specific to T1D to improve T1D management and decrease family conflict with immediate goals of improving family communication, achieving target glucose, and preventing acute and long-term T1D-related complications.[84,85]

The Family Teamwork intervention,[84] designed for adolescents and their caregivers, was tested by being delivered across multiple sessions by trained behavioral interventionists around the time of routine T1D medical appointments. Family Teamwork focuses on T1D education in the context of adolescent development, the importance of continued family involvement in T1D care across adolescence, improving family communication about T1D care, and preventing or reducing T1D-specific conflict. Family Teamwork interventions result in consistent, lasting effects on T1D outcomes, including improvements in A1C, family functioning, and quality of life.[84,86] One specific aspect of the Family Teamwork intervention approach is encouraging consistent parent-adolescent review of glucose data, which has a positive effect on glucose monitoring and reduced family conflict.[86]

Behavioral family systems therapy for diabetes comprises four components: problem-solving training, communication training, cognitive restructuring, and functional–structural family therapy.[85-87] Problem-solving methods encourage youth and parents to work together to define a problem clearly, identify possible solutions, and select the solution that they think will work best. Within a problem-solving framework, there are many approaches to collaborative defining of a problem (e.g., IDEAL [identify, describe, explore, anticipate, look back]) and setting a goal and implementing solutions to achieve it (e.g., SMART [specific, measurable, achievable, relevant, and time-bound]). Communication skills training involves establishing ground rules for acceptable and unacceptable verbal and nonverbal communication; providing instructions, feedback, and modeling; and rehearsing. Cognitive restructuring involves T1D- and family-specific maladaptive thoughts and attitudes. Functional–structural family therapy addresses challenges such as misaligned caregiver approaches to T1D management.[87] Participation in 10 sessions of behavioral family systems therapy for diabetes resulted in decreased family conflict, with gains maintained for up 18 months after treatment and reductions in A1C.[87]

In addition to these two multisession behavioral intervention protocols, there is some evidence that adults recognizing teen's T1D-related strengths and offering praise and reinforcement for what they are doing well for their T1D care may benefit psychosocial functioning.[88,89] Mental health professionals serve an essential role in helping parents and youth establish a routine of setting aside time each week to review T1D management tasks and glucose patterns together, in a nonjudgmental manner, focused on recognizing the hard work youth put into their T1D self-management and addressing any challenges they encounter (e.g., "How can I help?" "Let's figure this out together.").[88,90]

Most behavioral interventions in pediatric T1D have been developed and tested among primarily non-Hispanic White families with private health insurance who receive diabetes care at well-resourced academic medical center diabetes clinics.[91] Although this aligns with the prevalence of T1D among White children, rates of T1D in other populations are increasing, and the studied approaches and results may not apply directly to all children with T1D and their families. More research is needed into behavioral interventions for different racial and ethnic groups and families with fewer resources; in practice, mental health professionals must draw on their training in culturally appropriate care to tailor interventions to the families presenting for care.

Chapter 4 Worksheets

What goes in your kit?

_____'s T1D Kit

insulin

my t1d team

Name:
Role:

Name:
Role:

Name:
Role:

Name:
Role:

Name:
Role:

Setting SMART Diabetes Management Goals

S
Specific

What will you focus on changing? Who will be involved? Where/when will this take place?

M
Measurable

How much? How many? How will you know you completed your goal?

A
Achievable

Is there anything you need before you can work on your goal? Are there any barriers to your goal?

R
Relevant

Why is this goal important to you?

T
Time-bound

When will you start? When is the end date for this goal?

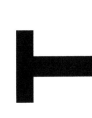

Problem-Solving Steps for Diabetes Management Challenges

What is the problem? _____

_____

_____

List solutions, consider + and - for each, and circle the one you want to try!

1.

2.

3.

4.

5.

Plan for trying solution. How will family/friends help you? When will you try it? What could get in the way?

_____

_____

_____

_____

The IDEAL Way to Problem Solve Diabetes Management Challenges

I	IDENTIFY THE PROBLEM

D	DEFINE EACH ASPECT OF PROBLEM

E	EXPLORE POSSIBLE SOLUTIONS AND POTENTIAL CONSEQUENCES AND OUTCOMES

A	ACT ON THE SOLUTION YOU CHOOSE

L	LOOK BACK. ARE YOU HAPPY WITH RESULTS? IF NOT- TRY ANOTHER SOLUTION!

Problem-Solving and SMART Goal-Setting for Diabetes Management Challenges

Describe the Problem:

What is your goal? Ideally, create a SMART goal that is Specific, Measurable, Achievable, Relevant, and Time-related.

What are barriers to achieving your goal? What gets in the way?

What are some possible solutions for achieving your goal?

Adapted from Nezu, Nezu, & D'Zurilla (2013). *Problem-Solving Therapy: A treatment manual.* NY, NY: Springer.

Problem-Solving Diabetes Challenges Using Pros and Cons

Solution	Pros (+)	Cons (-)
1.		
2.		
3.		

Which one do you want to try?

How did it work?

Adapted from Nezu, Nezu, & D'Zurilla (2013). *Problem-Solving Therapy: A treatment manual.* NY, NY: Springer.

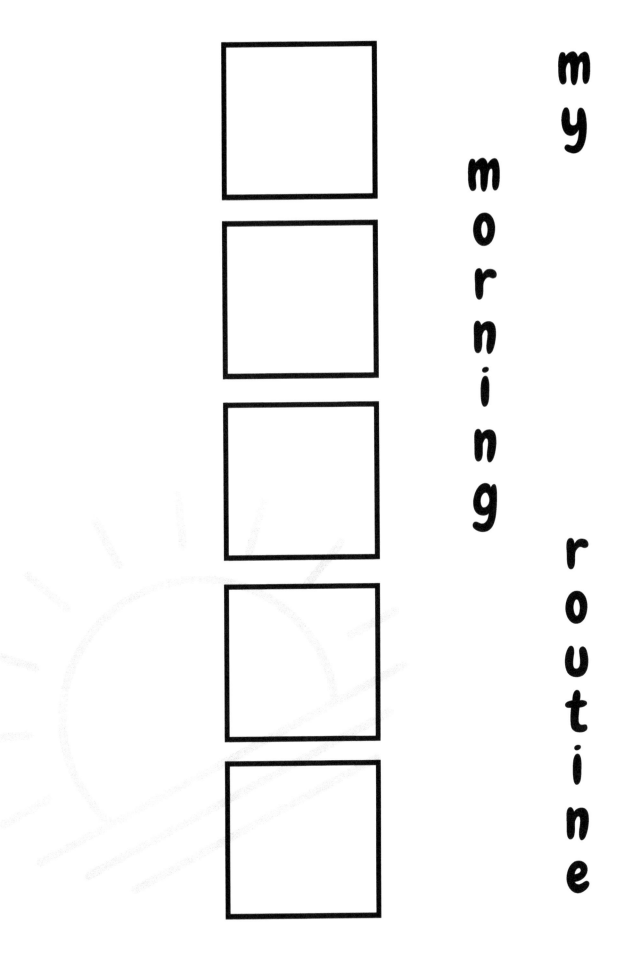

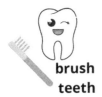
eat breakfast

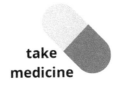
take medicine

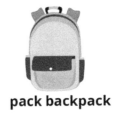
pack backpack

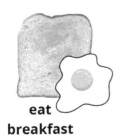
brush teeth

clean up

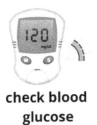
check blood glucose

shower

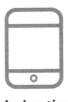
choice time

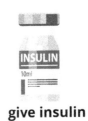
give insulin

get dressed

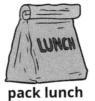
pack lunch

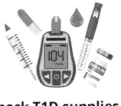
pack T1D supplies

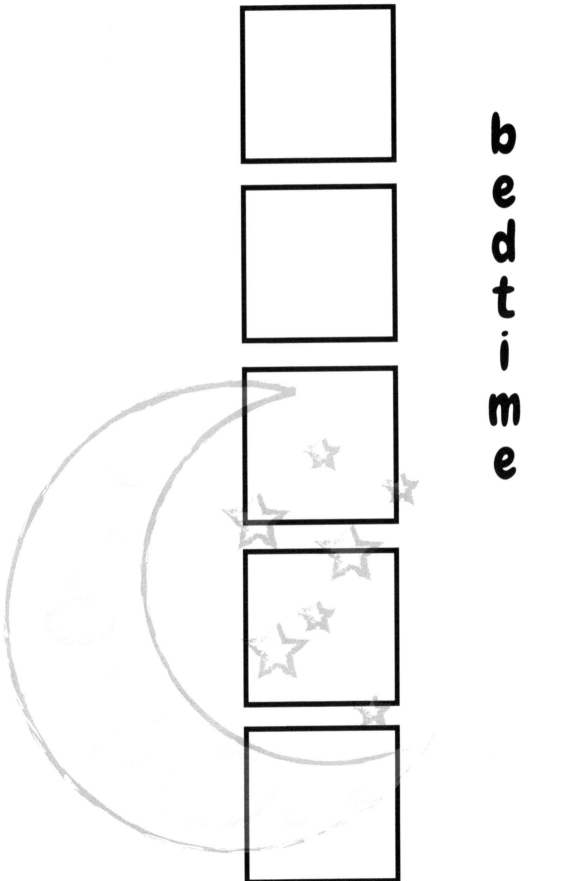

my bedtime routine

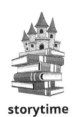

storytime

cuddle

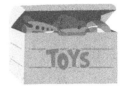

quiet play

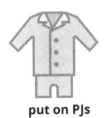

put on PJs

eat dinner

eat a snack

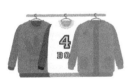

pick clothes for
tomorrow

put homework in
backpack

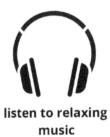

listen to relaxing
music

bathtime

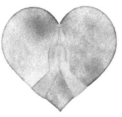

nighttime prayer
or gratitude

check blood
glucose

MY ROUTINE

NOTES:

MONDAY	TUESDAY	WEDNESDAY	THURSDAY	FRIDAY	SATURDAY	SUNDAY

MY MORNING ROUTINE

NOTES:

MONDAY	TUESDAY	WEDNESDAY	THURSDAY	FRIDAY	SATURDAY	SUNDAY

MY EVENING ROUTINE

NOTES:

MONDAY	TUESDAY	WEDNESDAY	THURSDAY	FRIDAY	SATURDAY	SUNDAY

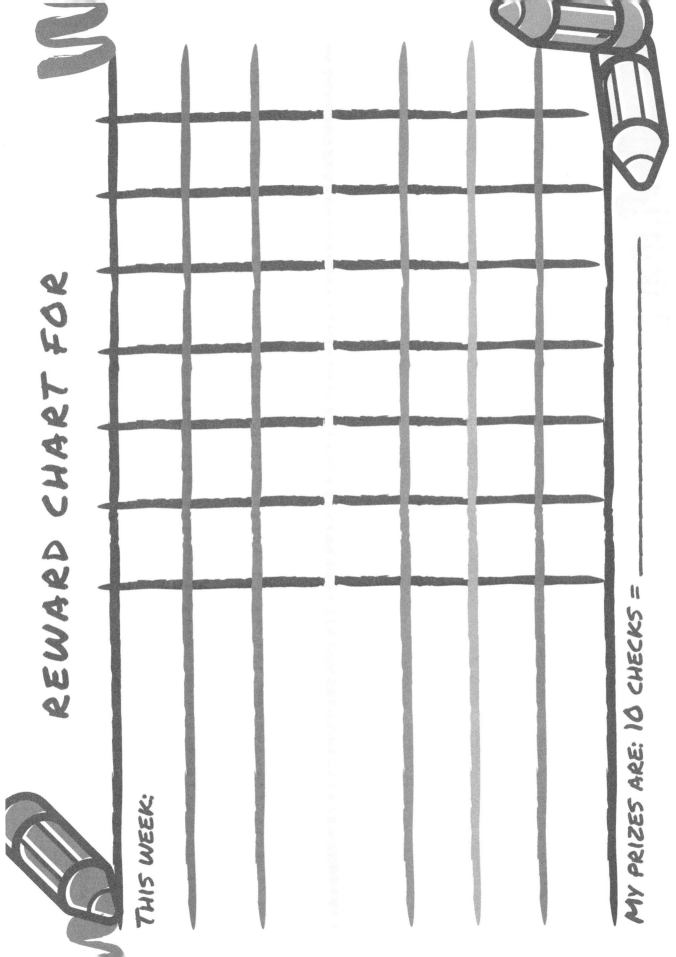

REWARD CHART FOR

THIS WEEK:

MY PRIZES ARE: 10 CHECKS = _____

Chapter 5
Emotions Associated with T1D

Many aspects of T1D, including glycemic variability throughout the day can trigger negative emotions.
A particularly difficult aspect of blood glucose variability is physiologic mood symptoms that mimic depressed mood, such as irritability, lethargy, and difficulty concentrating, in addition to frustration and worry. Other negative emotions related to high or low blood glucose include frustration, self-blame, and failure.

T1D devices were developed to help a person manage glucose, but they may be perceived by some youth to be burdensome because of the constant need to carry supplies. Other sources of burden include painful site changes, need to refill or replace supplies, device malfunctions, and sleep disruptions.[91,92] Many children feel self-conscious about wearing devices, especially when they are visible on the body, with increased feelings of stigma occurring for some individuals with T1D.[93,94] Children and parents may feel like their lives "revolve around T1D," which can lead to diabetes distress, burnout, depression, and anxiety (see the *Mood concerns and T1D* chapter).[95-98] Difficulties managing emotions are associated with suboptimal self-management,[99-101] glycemic variability,[100] and higher A1C.[102] Developing coping strategies to manage emotions in response to T1D demands promotes better quality of life and T1D outcomes. In addition, negative emotions about T1D extend beyond the person with T1D to family members, and may increase A1C.[103]

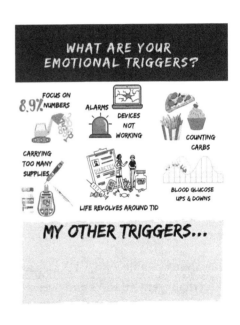

Common Emotional Responses in Youth

Isolation and Stigma

Many children and adolescents feel different from friends, classmates, and family members. Those who do not know other people with T1D or are the only student who needs to visit the school nurse for blood glucose checks or insulin delivery may feel isolated or alone. This may be particularly common in youth from racially and ethnically minoritized groups, given their lower rates of T1D prevalence and lower access to and engagement in T1D social outlets such as camp.[65,104]

Stigma associated with T1D includes feelings of rejection, exclusion, or blame related to having T1D,[94] and is often experienced as intrusive or judgmental comments from others, thereby creating anxiety in the person with T1D. People may make incorrect assumptions about the cause of T1D or make comments such as "Oh, you have diabetes, did you eat too much sugar?" Others may make inappropriate and hurtful jokes related to T1D, such as "Don't touch me, I don't want to get diabetes" or "I'd better not eat this cookie, I'll get diabetes." Some may confuse T1D with other diabetes types or reference relatives who have experienced complications from diabetes, such as "My grandmother has diabetes. She had to have her leg amputated last year." In these instances, individuals may be trying to relate by sharing their limited experience with diabetes; however, these comments can be frightening, hurtful, and isolating for the child with T1D or their parents.

Denial

Many children want to be like their peers who do not have T1D. It is common for young people with T1D, especially shortly after diagnosis and during periods of high stress, to hide or keep their T1D a secret or pretend they do not have it. In some cases, this may be developmentally appropriate and part of adjusting to living with T1D. However, not telling others about T1D is maladaptive and can be dangerous if self-management tasks are avoided or if there is no one to recognize and assist with a T1D-related emergency such as a severe hypoglycemic event.[105]

Anger and Resentment

Young people with T1D may feel angry at their parents, caregivers, and healthcare providers who conduct management tasks and oversee treatment, particularly if restrictions are placed on everyday activities due to T1D (e.g., limiting access to sweet foods) or oversight is perceived as intrusive, overbearing, or oppressive. Some children, especially older adolescents, may also resent feeling monitored by or dependent on others, and caregivers may resent the burden of T1D.[95]

Strategies to Navigate Emotional Responses to T1D

"Taking the emotion out of T1D" is a powerful strategy to help manage emotional responses to the challenges of living with T1D. As discussed in the *Language and communication about T1D* chapter, one strategy is to help children and parents avoid emotionally laden words like "good" and "bad" when discussing glucose numbers and reframe them as helpful numbers rather than as a performance evaluation or grade received. Mental health professionals can also guide children and parents to shift away from negative evaluative thoughts about glucose numbers (e.g., "What did my teen do/not do to get this awful number?") toward information-oriented thoughts (e.g., "I am glad to know these numbers—they provide information to help me figure out what to do to keep my child healthy" or " I'm disappointed to see this number isn't where I want it to be, but I know what to do to bring it up/down"). Reframing negative evaluations reduces the emotional burden of T1D and focuses attention on T1D management actions that should be taken next. Mental health professionals can also work with youth and their family members to reframe "diabetes failures"—such as "I am a failure for not being able to control my diabetes better"—into opportunities to take action. It can be helpful to examine a day in small increments of time to avoid evaluating the entire day as "good" or "bad." Instead, children and their parents can be taught to approach each blood glucose number and type of food eaten as a chance to learn how one's body works and figure out a way to engage differently with T1D.

Strategies to Manage Emotional Responses to T1D

T1D Event	Parent Concern	Parent Reaction	Youth Reaction	Strategy
Youth's blood glucose is low or really high	Youth is not treating the blood glucose	Repeated texting and/or calling	Annoyed, especially if ate snack or gave insulin	If youth does not respond in 5 min, parent contacts youth's friend
Youth's A1C is higher than expected	Long-term complications	Disappointment, frustration, anger	Helplessness, disappointment, anger	Do not talk about T1D on the way home; schedule a time later to discuss
Youth is irritable because blood glucose is high	Youth won't ever be able to manage self when high	Yells and tells youth to calm down	Youth becomes more irritable and uncooperative	Do not engage; walk away and wait until parent and youth can speak calmly
Youth's lows interfere with baseball	Youth might not be able to cope	Lectures youth about need to accept lows	Frustration	Develop coping skills (e.g., listening to music)

Chapter 5 Worksheets

WHAT ARE YOUR EMOTIONAL TRIGGERS?

FOCUS ON NUMBERS

9%

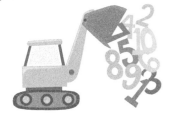

ALARMS

DEVICES NOT WORKING

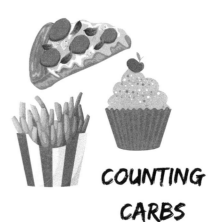

COUNTING CARBS

CARRYING TOO MANY SUPPLIES

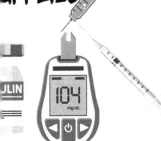

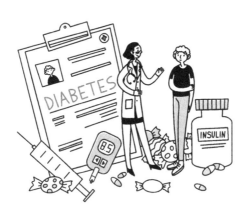

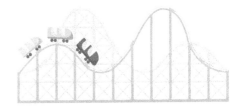

BLOOD GLUCOSE UPS & DOWNS

LIFE REVOLVES AROUND T1D

MY OTHER TRIGGERS...

Chapter 6
Mood Concerns and T1D

People with T1D are at increased risk of experiencing depression and distress. The healthcare professional working with children with T1D should be prepared to assess for and recommend strategies to manage these concerns.

Depression

Approximately 20% of children with T1D experience depressive symptoms, which is higher than the rate in their peers without T1D.[106] There may be a biological link between depression and diabetes.[107,108] Depressive symptoms may serve as a significant barrier to T1D self-management and are associated with multiple negative T1D health outcomes.[109-117] Specific symptoms of depression, such as low mood and energy, fatigue, and lack of motivation, may interfere with one's desire or ability to engage in self-management behaviors. Both low and high blood glucose may also cause an individual with T1D to feel unmotivated or physically unwell, potentially negatively affecting mood and interfering with engagement in T1D self-management behaviors. Because of overlap in symptom presentation, it may be difficult to distinguish the presence of a depressive disorder from depressive symptoms due to chronically high blood glucose. Mental health providers should always consider glucose values and trends when assessing, diagnosing, and treating individuals with T1D who present with depressive symptoms.

Diabetes Distress

Diabetes distress is a reaction to the everyday, ongoing challenges, demands, and relentlessness of living with T1D.[118] In contrast to depression, diabetes distress involves negative feelings specific to diabetes. Emotional and behavioral aspects of diabetes distress include diabetes-specific burnout, anger, frustration, stress, worry, and negativity, as well as feeling misunderstood by providers, friends, and family members.[119] Approximately 33% of adolescents with T1D experience diabetes distress, which may occur with or independent of depression.[120] Diabetes distress is often linked with higher A1C[120] and lower engagement in self-management behaviors.[120] Whereas diabetes distress is common across the pediatric T1D population, young children from racially and ethnically minoritized groups and those with low socioeconomic status are more likely to experience diabetes distress.[121] Elevated diabetes distress as well as glycemic disparities in these groups highlight the need for culturally appropriate mental health care.

Related to diabetes distress is diabetes burnout, an experience that is characterized by feeling extremely frustrated and discouraged by T1D or being "sick and tired of T1D." Individuals with T1D describe burnout as mental and physical exhaustion, feeling disconnected from others and themselves and diabetes care, and a sense of being powerless to overcome T1D-related stress.[120] Diabetes burnout is common and it often waxes and wanes;[120] preventing or minimizing its impact helps maintain the child's engagement in T1D self-management tasks and potentially prevents increasing A1C.

Acknowledging an individual's successes with T1D is one strategy to reduce the risk for burnout. Additional strategies to promote resilience and prevent burnout include focusing on what the child with T1D is doing well, acknowledging how the family has successfully worked together to manage T1D, or working to recognize other strengths family members have developed.[122,123]

Whereas some people may struggle to identify positive aspects of diabetes, many people who have T1D are able to identify strengths and successes, and youth often appreciate when parents notice positive actions associated with T1D self-management.[89]

Treating Depression and Diabetes Distress

Depression and diabetes distress are treated similarly. An important first step of any treatment plan related to mood is to reduce chronically elevated blood glucose by working closely with T1D medical providers to address hyperglycemia. Several evidence-based interventions for depression, including problem-solving skills therapy, interpersonal therapy, or acceptance and commitment therapy, along with cognitive behavioral therapy, can be adapted to focus on T1D-specific concerns that contribute to or exacerbate mood symptoms. Interventions to target diabetes distress are specifically focused on the particular stressors and burdens related to T1D that youth or parents experience. In addition, the evidence-based Penn Resiliency Program[124] adapted for T1D[123] reduces symptoms of depression or diabetes distress in adolescents from 14–18 years of age.

CBT: Depression and T1D	
Psychoeducation	• How blood glucose fluctuations affect mood. • Bidirectional relationship between low mood and less engagement in self-management behaviors.
Mood Tracking	• Incorporate blood glucose monitoring into mood tracking to raise awareness of link between mood and blood glucose.
Behavioral Activation	• Inactivity can affect insulin needs and blood glucose readings; increasing physical activity can lower blood glucose. • Monitor blood glucose and insulin needs in relation to physical activity changes.
Problem-Solving	• Set T1D-specific behavioral goals. Focus on self-management behaviors, not blood glucose numbers or A1C as the goal. • Use problem-solving to address barriers to implementing goals.
Relaxation Training	• Ensure blood glucose is stable and within target range to minimize disruptions to relaxation strategies.
Cognitive Restructuring	• Focus on thoughts and feelings about T1D. Restructure negative cognitions to focus on successes, capabilities, and supports related to T1D.

Suicide Risk

Young people with T1D are 61% more likely than their peers to report suicidal thoughts, with nearly 8%–15% endorsing suicidal ideation.[125-127] Youth with T1D have a 1.7-times higher risk than their peers for suicide attempts,[126] and 16% have made a suicide attempt.[127] Risk factors associated with a suicide attempt in the general young population include, but are not limited to, previous suicide attempts, mental health disorders such as depression, feelings of hopelessness, easy access to lethal methods of self-harm, and barriers to mental health care.[128]

According to the interpersonal theory of suicide, "thwarted belongingness" (feeling as if one does not fit in or is not understood) and "perceived burdensomeness" (thinking one's existence makes life harder or more stressful for family and friends) are two factors that contribute to suicidal ideation, especially when accompanied by feelings of hopelessness.[129,130] Two-thirds of children with T1D who report suicidal ideation feel they are a burden to their family, in part because of T1D and especially when there is family conflict.[127] Assessing perceived burdensomeness in children with T1D is especially important given the daily demands of its management and financial implications for families.

Suicidal thoughts occur on a continuum, and not everyone who reports a history of suicidal ideation is at imminent risk of self-harm. It is important to conduct a thorough assessment of past and current suicidal thoughts and death ideation (i.e., wanting to die but not taking action to effect death, the belief that one would be better off dead), intent to die by suicide, fear of death, plans and preparations to die by suicide, means to make an attempt, and family history of suicide.[131]

Mental health professionals must communicate clearly and recognize that asking about suicidal ideation is not going to "put the idea of suicide into someone's head" or increase the risk of suicide. Acknowledging and asking about suicidality may actually serve as a protective factor against a suicide attempt and may reduce suicidal ideation by providing a sense of support.[132,133] Identifying protective factors that

Essential Components of Suicide Risk	
Frequency/duration/intensity of current suicidal and death ideations	Frequency, duration, intensity of current non-suicidal self-injurious behaviors
History of suicidal and death ideations	History of non-suicidal self-injurious behaviors
Number of previous suicide attempts	Family history of suicide
Suicidal desire (0 = no desire at all to 10 = highest desire)	Feelings of thwarted belongingness and hopelessness
Suicidal intent (0 = no intent at all to 10 = highest intent)	Perceptions of being a burden
Preparations to make a suicide attempt	Capability for suicide
Plans to make a suicide attempt	Recent stressors
Access to lethal means	Mental health history (e.g., depression, impulsivity, risky behaviors, substance use, trauma, insomnia)

mitigate suicidal risk is essential when assessing suicide risk. Problem-solving skills and other adaptive coping skills, optimism, future orientation, reasons for living, positive family relationships, social connectedness, and supportive school environments are protective against suicidal behavior.[134,135]

Lethality of Insulin

Clinical management of suicide or death ideation in youth with T1D must include assessing and restricting access to means of self-harm, including insulin. Although insulin is medically necessary for peope with T1D, the difference between an appropriate dose of insulin and a potentially lethal overdose can be small.[136] Even a small amount of insulin could provide lethal means for suicide by inducing severe hypoglycemia in a short amount of time. Intentionally omitting insulin can also lead to a less immediate but still dangerous potential for diabetic ketoacidosis, which typically requires hospitalization and can lead to death if not treated promptly and appropriately.

Some people, particularly children or those new to T1D, may not be aware of the lethality of insulin. Thus, mental health professionals may need to exercise caution in assessing specific plans for suicide attempts as well as discussing means restriction with a child who has not suggested insulin as a potential method of intentional self-harm. As noted previously, asking children about suicide will not put the idea in their heads or increase risk,[132,133] but it is advisable to avoid introducing information about lethal means or methods of suicide to those who are already experiencing suicidal ideation or intent. When appropriate, mental health professionals may consider speaking with parents separately from children to discuss the potential risk of using insulin as a means of self-harm, which allows parents an opportunity to express a genuine reaction in the event they are just learning of their child's suicidal ideation and the opportunity to ask questions without censoring themselves in front of the child.

Given the lethality of insulin, restricting access to insulin in children with suicidal ideation may be required, which introduces unique challenges especially with older children, who may be accustomed to managing T1D without direct parental observation. Mental health professionals should help families determine how to ensure means restriction based on their circumstances. For youth taking multiple daily insulin injections using vials and syringes, means restriction is relatively clear—a parent or another adult (e.g., school nurse) should administer or monitor all insulin injections. Securing insulin in a medication lockbox, which can be stored where needed and for which a parent or another adult holds the key, is ideal. For youth who are engaged in activities outside the home and who need to take their insulin with them, families may develop a plan for safe administration and monitoring of insulin dosing. However, if assessment reveals concern for imminent risk of overdosing on insulin, the child may need more intensive supervision or mental health care until the risk is reduced or safety can be ensured, or both. For those using an insulin pump, there are additional challenges. Youth have constant and private access to the pump, which could make it easier to administer an overdose of insulin without an adult noticing. Parents and providers may want to consider whether an insulin pump can be used safely or if it would be advisable to use insulin injections, which can be more easily monitored and secured by an adult, until use of the pump is deemed safe. Mental health professionals should encourage parents to speak with their child's T1D care providers about this decision. If the child switches to using insulin injections, it

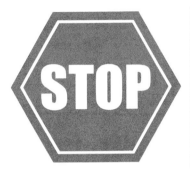

Discontinue pump immediately if...
- Active suicide ideation with intent and plan.
- Plan to attempt suicide with insulin overdose.
- Recently attempted suicide by any means and has not received mental health treatment since the attempt.
- Note: In these situations, referral to local hospital emergency center or inpatient mental health care is likely necessary.

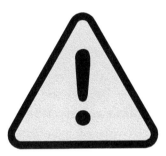

Likely need to remove pump and use insulin injections monitored by caregiver if...
- Recurrent or current suicide ideation with high intent, even if there is no plan or suicidal/self-harm behavior AND
- Youth cannot engage in meaningful safety planning OR
- Youth is not meeting weekly with mental health professional.

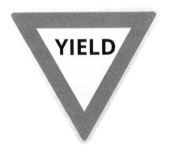

May be able to continue pump with close monitoring if...
- Intermittent suicide ideation but intent, plan, or behaviors AND
- Diabetes distress and perceived T1D burden is significantly lower with insulin pump AND
- Youth engages well in safety planning, including coping skills, people they can talk to in times of distress, and reasons to live AND
- Youth is receiving mental health treatment.

Can likely continue insulin pump if...
- There is a history of suicidal ideation or death ideation, but no current suicide ideation, plan or behaviors AND
- Youth engages well in safety planning, including coping skills, people they can talk to in times of distress, and reasons to live AND
- Caregivers are able to monitor blood glucoses and insulin administration on daily basis.

is recommended that mental health professionals, the T1D medical team, and parents frame this as an opportunity to increase safety and provide optimal support to the child—not as a punishment—while emphasizing that this solution is likely temporary. In the event of safety concerns and recommendations to restrict access to insulin, it is important that the mental health professional speak with the child's T1D care team (with permission) to understand potential safety risks and engage in discussion about the best choice for insulin administration based on the child's and family's situation.

Crisis Prevention or Safety Plans

Crisis prevention or safety planning helps identify triggers, coping skills, supports, means restriction, and reasons for living, thereby reducing risk of engagement in self-harm behaviors and increasing one's ability to manage suicidal thoughts when they occur.[137] Crisis prevention or safety planning should be a collaborative process among mental health professionals, the youth with T1D, and their parents. No-suicide contracts, in which individuals agree not to harm themselves regardless of their current ideation or intent, are not recommended: they do not reduce risk of suicide,[138] may be perceived negatively and disrupt the therapeutic alliance,[139] are not legally binding,[140] and may lead to litigation to determine liability.[141] Using collaborative crisis prevention and safety planning (two worksheets on safety planning and coping skills—one for children and the other for adolescents—are presented at the end of this chapter) results in faster reduction in suicidal ideation and reduced hospitalization rates relative to no-suicide contracts.[140]

Frequent reassessment of suicidal ideation and safety is recommended. Mental health providers should monitor whether 1) suicidal ideation has increased, 2) adjustments to the crisis prevention or safety plan are needed, 3) new safety concerns have arisen, and 4) current care is effective and appropriate. Reassessment helps mental health professionals monitor decreases in suicidal ideation and depressive symptoms, as well as improvements in coping, which aids planning for resuming or increasing independence for young people whose parents have increased daily involvement in T1D care tasks related to safety concerns.

Chapter 6 Worksheets

Child

Safety Plan & Coping Skills

What things can I do to help myself feel better?

Who can I talk to when I need help feeling better or if I feel unsafe?

Ways to make the environment safer.

How can I tell that I am getting very upset, sad, mad, or unsafe?

What are some things or people in my life that make me feel happy, loved, and safe? What things can I hope for in the future?

Suicide Prevention Lifeline:
1-800-273-8255

Crisis Text Line:
Text HOME to 741741

The Trevor Project Lifeline
(LBGTQ+ youth): 1-866-488-7386

Call 911

Teen/Young Adult

Safety Plan & Coping Skills

Coping Strategies. How can I distract myself when I feel unsafe?

People who can help me when I feel unsafe.

Ways to make the environment safer.

Reasons I want to be alive.

How can I tell I am feeling unsafe? List your thought, feelings, or situations.

Suicide Prevention Lifeline:
1-800-273-8255

Crisis Text Line:
Text HOME to 741741

The Trevor Project Lifeline
(LBGTQ+ youth): 1-866-488-7386

Call 911

Think-Feel-Do

Situation (what was happening):

's time for a pump site change.

Noooooooo! I don't want to.

Think

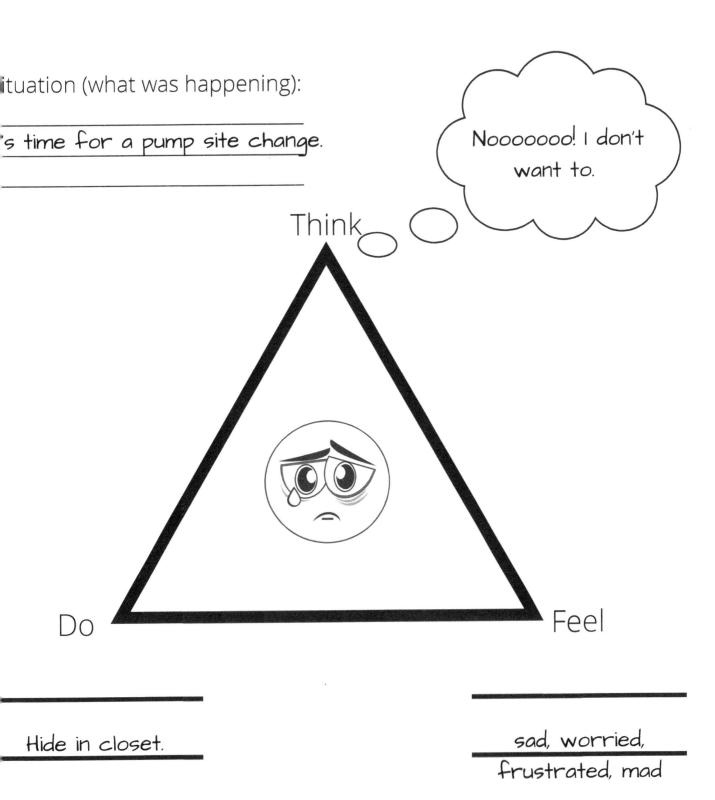

Do

Feel

Hide in closet.

sad, worried, frustrated, mad

Think-Feel-Do

tuation (what was happening):

My mom asked me if I had
checked blood glucose yet.

She never trusts
me. She thinks I am a
failure.

Think

Do

Feel

ie and tell her I did.

I her to leave me alone.

Worthless

Sad

Think-Feel-Do

ituation (what was happening):

_____

's time for a pump site change.

_____

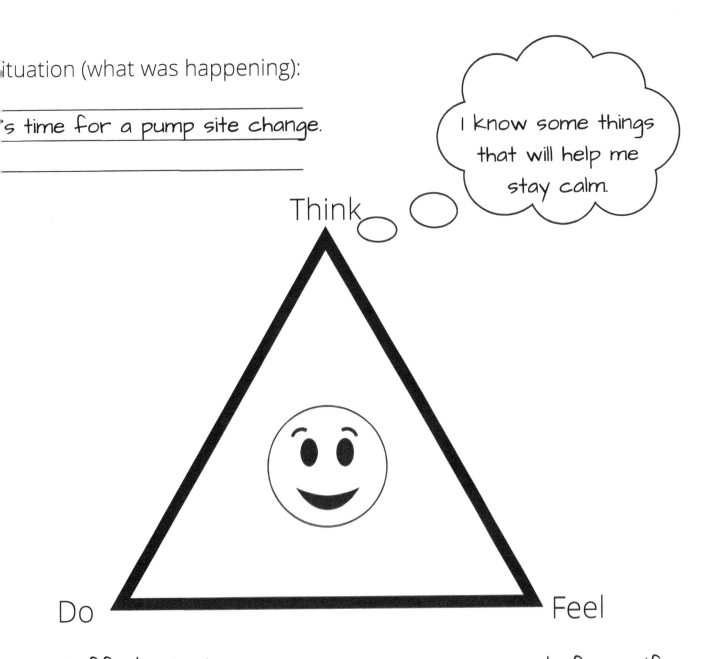

Think

I know some things that will help me stay calm.

Do

Feel

my stuffed animals
nd practice guided
magery while dad does
site change

proud of myself
for doing site
change without
crying

Think-Feel-Do

What could you think instead?

tuation (what was happening):

_____

_____

_____

Think

Do

Feel

_____
_____
_____

_____
_____
_____

Chapter 7
T1D-Related Worries and Anxiety

One-third of children with T1D experience anxiety related to specific aspects of living with T1D, including social anxiety, fear of hypoglycemia, anxiety related to uptake of new technology, and needle anxiety or avoidance.[142,143]

T1D-Specific Social Anxiety

Rates of social anxiety may be higher in young people with T1D[142] compared with their peers without T1D. Social anxiety in young people with T1D is often specifically related to social aspects of T1D, including others learning or knowing that the person has T1D, completing T1D-related tasks in front of other people or in public places, answering questions or talking about T1D, experiencing judgment about T1D, managing or communicating about T1D in dating situations, or having symptoms of hypoglycemia or hyperglycemia in front of other people.[142,143] Social anxiety disorder, in which youth experience anxiety in a wide range of social situations and diabetes-specific social anxiety may or may not co-occur.

It may be necessary to distinguish among clinically elevated anxiety, developmentally appropriate concerns about privacy, and secrecy. Privacy involves a preference to complete T1D-related tasks without an audience, or avoid attention from others, whereas secrecy involves actively hiding T1D and its management from others, which may negatively affect daily T1D self-management and well-being.[144] Youth may prefer privacy but be willing to complete T1D self-management tasks in the presence of others when necessary. To avoid the development of anxiety, young people with T1D may need to practice completing T1D-related tasks in the presence of others. People who experience high anxiety or who engage in secrecy likely delay or avoid engaging in T1D self-management tasks and may benefit from intervention to address concerns and behaviors that interfere with optimal T1D management. Treating T1D-specific social anxiety is important to minimize suboptimal T1D outcomes and improve quality of life.[142] Treatment for social anxiety disorder and T1D-specific social anxiety both respond best to cognitive behavioral therapy with exposure and response prevention.

Fear of Hypoglycemia

Hypoglycemia is a common source of anxiety in children with T1D and their parents given the significant and negative health outcomes that may occur, especially those associated with severe hypoglycemia. Many of the physical sensations commonly associated with hypoglycemia mimic physical sensations of intense anxiety and panic, such as dizziness and rapid heart rate. If children repeatedly experience these physical sensations paired with hypoglycemia and anxiety, they may develop fear of hypoglycemia[145]

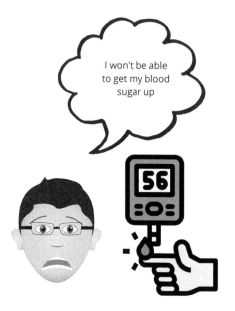

through classical conditioning. Moreover, the overlap in symptoms between hypoglycemic episodes and intense anxiety make it difficult to differentiate the cause of physical symptoms. Thus, children may start to feel anxiety when their blood glucose begins to decrease even if it is not yet near being classified as a low blood glucose. Fear of hypoglycemia in its severe presentation is akin to a specific phobia of a low blood glucose.

Some fear of hypoglycemia is adaptive because it serves as a warning to children with T1D or their parents about the real risks associated with severe low blood glucose and may motivate them to engage in T1D self-management behaviors to prevent or treat hypoglycemia. Fear of hypoglycemia is problematic when it compromises quality of life or T1D self-management. Impairing fear of hypoglycemia may present even in the absence of having experienced an actual severe hypoglycemic event, suggesting that treating fear of hypoglycemia requires intense fear management.[146]

Traditional T1D education is not likely to help individuals with T1D or their parents manage fear of hypoglycemia. Evidence-based intervention is essential to address fear of hypoglycemia not only due to the psychological distress it causes but also because maintaining hyperglycemia as a coping strategy for managing severe fear of hypoglycemia is a significant barrier to achieving optimal A1C.

Although questionnaires to assess fear of hypoglycemia are useful for screening symptoms,[147–150] a comprehensive clinical interview about hypoglycemia-related worries is the gold standard and is more informative for clinical treatment planning. Individuals with T1D and their parents often habituate to their worry about low blood glucoses and the behaviors they engage in (e.g., excessively checking blood glucose), which become their "normal" experience. Thus, nuanced and specific questioning may be needed to ascertain whether someone recognizes that his or her

CBT for Fear of Hypoglycemia

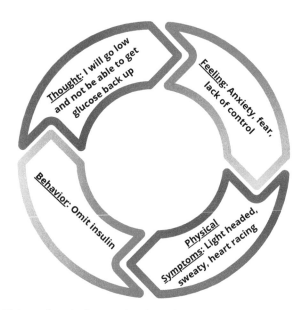

This cycle reinforces the thoughts that it is not safe to give prescribed amount of insulin. A vicious cycle of anxiety and avoidance occurs.

worry about hypoglycemia is maladaptive and impairing.

Graduated exposure therapy and cognitive behavioral therapy with exposure and response prevention, an evidence-based approach to treating anxiety, is suggested as treatment for impairing fear of hypoglycemia.[146] This approach has been implemented successfully in clinical care[151] and is being tested in randomized clinical trials.[152,153] Preliminary data suggest that exposure and response prevention is likely successful in treating fear of hypoglycemia, reducing symptoms of generalized anxiety, and improving blood glucoses without increasing hypoglycemia episodes. Treatment involves normalizing the fear response, identifying current strategies for managing fear (e.g., avoiding in-range blood glucose), providing psychoeducation, determining a perceived "safe" blood glucose value (i.e., the blood glucose number that a person feels is "safe," thereby guaranteeing that a low blood glucose will not happen; for example, some

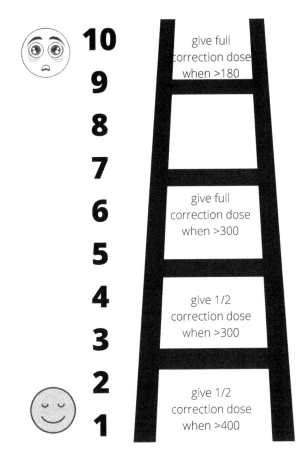

people will only give insulin for blood glucose values >250 mg/dL), and using graduated exposure with response prevention to help the child move slowly from his or her "safe" blood glucose range to the in-target range,[146,152,153] while helping the individual with T1D and/or their parents manage the anxiety that may be triggered by this process (see the fear of hypoglycemia worksheets, including the "Fear of hypoglycemia graph" to ascertain degree of worry in comparison with degree of vigilance, "Cognitive behavioral therapy for fear of hypoglycemia," "Fear of hypoglycemia math exercise," "Fear of hypoglycemia cognition cartoon," and "Fear ladder" [to be used with any T1D-related anxiety]).

Sample Interview Questions for Assessing Fear of Hypoglycemia

These questions can also be addressed to the child's parents to assess their anxieties around hypoglycemia.

- What did your T1D provider tell you is the target range for your blood glucose?
- Many individuals have a blood glucose number where they feel most comfortable. Do you have a number like this? What is the number during the day? What about before bed? What about during the night?
- Is there a certain blood glucose number that you prefer not to correct during the day? At night?
- What blood glucose number do you consider to be low? Do you usually treat that number by eating? If so, what would you eat?
- Do you eat a snack before bed? If so, how many grams of carbohydrate are in the snack? Is there a certain blood glucose number at which you always have a snack before bed? Is there a blood glucose number at which you would not have a snack before bed?
- Do you take insulin if the glucose before bed is 180? (Query increasing blood glucose values: What about 190? What about 200?).
- Do you ever reduce the amount of insulin you take? If yes, in what situations? Before bed?
- Do you ever second-guess the amount of insulin the insulin pump tells you to give?
- Do you ever give less than the recommended dose of insulin the pump tells you to give? If yes, in what situations? Before bed?
- Do you ever omit giving insulin because you are worried the blood glucose will go too low? When do you do that?
- Do you ever suspend insulin in the pump because you are worried the blood glucose will go too low? When do you do that?
- When your blood glucose is low, do you eat 15 g of carbohydrate, wait 15 minutes, and recheck? If not, what do you to eat in response to a low glucose? Is it ever the case that so many grams of carbohydrate are eaten that there is then a "rebound" high (>300 mg/dL)?
- How many times do you get up in the night to check blood glucose or the continuous glucose monitor? Do you wake up naturally or do you set alarms?
- How many times a day do you check your blood glucose with a fingerstick? What about at night?
- Do you only give insulin when eating? Do you ever cover the carbohydrate intake while not correcting for a high blood glucose? Do you ever avoid carbohydrate intake to avoid covering it with insulin?
- Do you worry about the pump giving too much insulin? Do you have concerns that it will malfunction and give too much insulin, and that you might die?
- Do you worry about whether the continuous glucose monitor is accurate? Do you ever think that it is not accurate? If so, when?
- Do you ever take a break from the continuous glucose monitor because the constant number of readings is overwhelming and creates anxiety?

- Have you ever stopped using the continuous glucose monitor completely because the constant number of readings was overwhelming and created anxiety?
- Do you ever think that you are more sensitive to insulin than usual or compared with others? When have you thought this?
- Do you ever think that your blood glucose will drop at any time? When have you thought this?
- Do you ever think that your blood glucose will continue to drop even if it has been treated? When have you thought this?
- Do you ever think that your blood glucose drops rapidly during the night? When have you thought this?
- Do you ever think that you will have a seizure? When have you thought this?
- Do you ever think that you will have a critically low blood glucose and nobody will be there to help? When have you thought this?
- Do you ever think that it is better for your blood glucose to run high than to risk having a critically low blood glucose?
- For parents: If you have a sharing app, how many times a day do you check it to see what your child's blood glucose is? How many times per hour? Is this different in the day versus the night?

Using the fear of hypoglycemia math exercise to highlight low blood glucoses that have occurred in the context of all of the blood glucoses that have been measured throughout one's T1D duration may be helpful.

Let's bring down worry!
A little mathematics exercise!

A	Number of days Johnny has had T1D...	700
B	Number of lows Johnny has had...	575
C	Number of lows for which Johnny has needed assistance...	1
D	Number of lows where Johnny has needed assistance / total blood glucose checks Johnny has done...	=1/ 575= .002%

What does all this mean?
These data show us that Johnny VERY RARELY has a low when he needs assistance. We also know Johnny has NEVER had a severe low where he needed glucagon. The chances that Johnny will have a severe low are...VERY LOW.

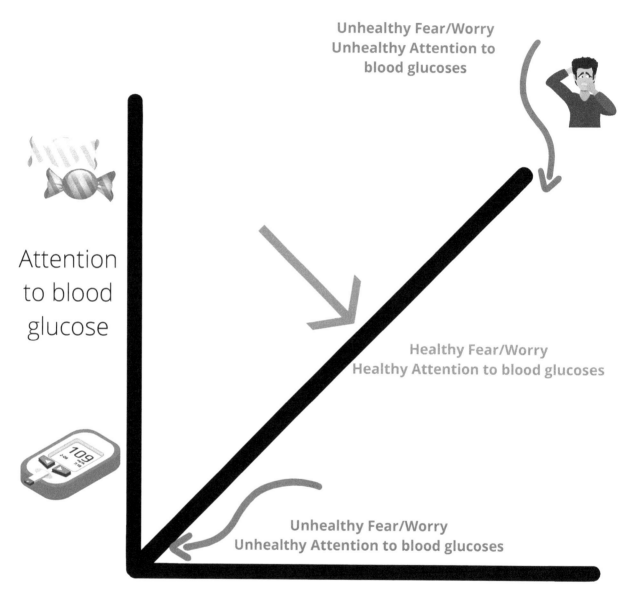

Where do you fall on the graph?

Hypoglycemia Unawareness

Individuals with T1D, especially those with lower A1C, may have relatively reduced physical awareness of fluctuations in their glucose. This can be particularly dangerous and anxiety-provoking if an individual loses the ability to sense when they are hypoglycemic. Blood glucose awareness training is a manualized approach to help adults with T1D regain their ability to detect fluctuations in glucoses,[154] which has been adapted to be administered online (blood glucose training at home). The intervention has only been examined in adults with T1D.

Needle Anxiety and Blood Phobia in Individuals with T1D

The negative physiologic response to having a needle injected into the skin or seeing blood is common and (in most cases) adaptive, and needle fear is common.[155-157] Therefore, it is normal for young people with T1D, especially younger children and people who have had little exposure to needles or blood, to have some degree of distress, fear, or anxiety with needle injections or blood draws.[158,159] However, some children have significant fears and may avoid blood glucose checks, adminstering insulin injections, device insertions, or routine bloodwork. Needle anxiety is very common in children and adolescents with T1D.[158,159] Although many individuals resolve their needle anxiety or avoidance relatively quickly through repeated exposure to the T1D treatment demands, some experience persistent fear that may develop into needle phobia symptoms.[158,159]

Needle anxiety or fear of blood in young people with T1D may result in avoidance of blood glucose checks, fewer insulin injections, delays in changing diabetes technology infusion sets, reluctance to complete routine laboratory blood draws, and avoidance of rotating areas of the finger for blood glucose monitoring, or areas of the body when changing insulin pump infusion sets and continuous glucose monitoring sensors. For those who do not rotate sites, scar tissue may form at the fingertips or build up under the skin (i.e., lipohypertrophy), which interferes with insulin absorption. Engagement in these behaviors often leads to higher A1C,[159] but needle anxiety or fear of blood are not readily recognized by medical providers as a potential reason for low engagement in T1D self-management.[156]

Mental health professionals must distinguish the type and severity of needle anxiety or fear of blood that children experience, identifying fear (a 'fight-or-flight' reaction [the sympathetic nervous system response that drives the body into action when feeling threatened] in the immediate moment), anxiety (negative emotions in anticipation of a needle experience), or phobia (combination of both fear and anxiety that is disproportionately high compared with the actual danger that the specific situation or object poses).[155] Assessments for needle anxiety or avoidance should include gathering information about the child's typical behavioral responses to the feared stimulus, as ~25% also experience loss of consciousness or fainting, which requires a different treatment approach than fight-or-light responses.[156,160] Strategies used to manage pain associated with injections (i.e., distraction) are contraindicated and may interfere with progress when extinguishing needle- or blood-related anxieties.[160] There are few case studies[161] on needle phobia interventions specific to young people with T1D. Therefore, most recommendations for treating needle anxiety or phobias in young people with T1D are derived from the general needle anxiety clinical guidelines, which have a strong evidence base for those >7 years of age and are likely to have a similar positive effect for all ages.[160]

Excessive fear of needles or blood may be 1) a learned response from previous negative interactions, 2) a learned response from a parent's modeling of his or her own fears, or 3) due to anticipatory fear of losing consciousness or fainting. For youth who have developed needle anxiety or avoidance or fear of blood due to a conditioned/learned response (i.e., not from loss of consciousness or fainting), cognitive behavioral therapy with exposure and response prevention is recommended.[146,160] For those who lose consciousness or faint in response to needles or laboratory blood draws, applied muscle tension strategies should be used to keep blood pressure and heart rate elevated to minimize the potential for loss of consciousness or fainting.

Treating T1D-Related Worries and Anxiety

Cognitive behavioral therapy with exposure and response prevention, which are effective, evidence-based treatments for anxiety, can be adapted and applied to treat T1D-specific anxiety. Treatment generally begins with psychoeducation about anxiety and the role of avoidance in maintaining and increasing anxiety across time. Discuss with the family that the goal of treatment is to help children face their fears in a gradual manner, which allows them to build confidence and learn that anxiety need not interfere with taking care of their health and having good quality of life. Then, explain how thoughts and feelings relate to behaviors, with a focus on T1D-related examples of each. Teach children to identify early signs of anxiety in their thoughts (e.g., worries, self-talk) and their body (e.g., increased heart rate, faster breathing). It is important to help youth recognize how high or low glucoses affect their thoughts and feelings, and how those thoughts and feelings then affect their T1D self-management behaviors.

The child should be helped to identify common "thinking traps" and apply the concept to T1D-specific worries and anxiety. For example, individuals with T1D and anxiety may engage in catastrophizing, whereby a discrete thought (e.g., "I might have a high blood sugar") grows into a pressing fear (e.g., "My continuous glucose monitor alarm will go off, I'll have to get up in the middle of class, and everyone will look at me and think I'm weird"). Some may engage in mind-reading, in which individuals make assumptions, usually negative, about what others are thinking (e.g., "The people at the restaurant looked at me when I injected my insulin—they must be grossed out or think I'm doing drugs"). Helping youth identify these thinking traps is an important step toward modifying maladaptive thoughts to be less influential. Some children may also benefit from learning relaxation exercises, such as diaphragmatic breathing, mindfulness, or grounding exercises to use when they experience these anxious thoughts. Sessions focused on cognitive- and relaxation-based coping skills may be helpful for youth with a wider range of anxious thoughts or who need more support before beginning exposures. However, some children may be able to move directly from psychoeducation into graduated exposures. Given the relationship between emotional distress and variations in glucose, children and parents should be advised to monitor glucose when they notice changes in emotions or behavior and treat highs or lows as needed.

As mentioned in the section on fear of hypoglycemia, the foundation treatment for T1D-specific anxiety involves exposure and response prevention, in which a hierarchy or "fear ladder" is built and then practiced. Fear ladder items that can be cut out and placed on the ladder are found in this section and include items pertaining to answering questions about T1D, finding out about the T1D, performing T1D-related tasks in public, and having a high or low glucose occur while in public. A worksheet is also included about assigned exposures for homework and identifying coping strategies when practicing them (see the "Practicing exposures" worksheet).

Mental health providers help children gradually move up the ladder, facing fears of increasing intensity while preventing behaviors that may interfere with fully confronting his or her anxiety. When building a hierarchy focused on T1D-specific anxiety, it is important to develop a wide range of activities targeting the child's specific fears and identify tasks that are appropriate for each of the ladder steps using subjective units of distress ratings or a "fear thermometer."

Ultimately, the goals of T1D-related anxiety treatment are to help youth with T1D learn that 1) the feared stimulus is not likely to cause the serious harm that they anticipate and 2) their distress experienced during the exposure can be tolerated.[146,160] Treatment often includes the following components:

1. Psychoeducation will help the child understand how avoidance of the feared stimulus (e.g., needles or blood from laboratory draws) is counterproductive.

2. Direct anxiety management strategies (e.g., deep breathing, biofeedback, progressive muscle relaxation) are used to counter fight-or-flight physiologic responses. Other anxiety reduction strategies, such as distraction, should be minimized because they serve as a form of avoidance and prevent the child from learning a new response to the feared stimulus.

3. Cognitive restructuring strategies are used to help youth identify negative thoughts and restructure them into more accurate representations of the actual risk.

4. A fear hierarchy from least to most fearful stimuli (e.g., picture of a needle → injecting into oranges → going to a laboratory) is created with the young person, who is then exposed to the item represented at the lowest step of the hierarchy until the physiologic arousal response (e.g., elevated heart rate) decreases, with the child moving up the list as anxiety over each item is resolved. This stepwise approach may require several sessions as the child builds confidence until he or she reaches full exposure. A more rapid alternative is *in vivo* exposure directly to the most feared stimulus.

5. Addressing parental anxiety (especially for younger children) is important because parental fear modeling can affect how children experience needles and laboratory blood draws.[160] Parents should be coached to provide effective reassurances (i.e., use of humor or nonprocedural talk instead of "Don't worry") during exposures.[160]

Chapter 7 Worksheets

CBT for Fear of Hypoglycemia

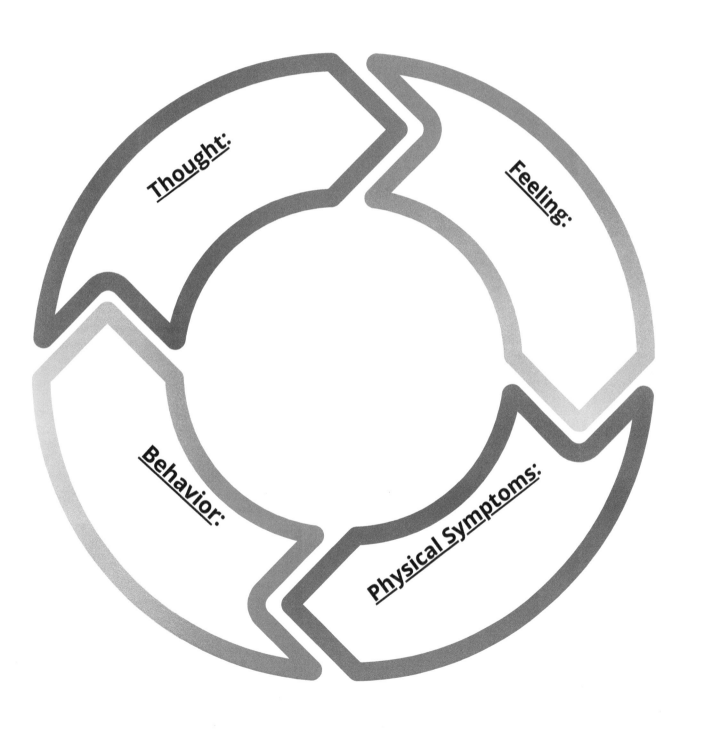

Thought:

Feeling:

Behavior:

Physical Symptoms:

Challenging Unhelpful Thoughts

Automatic Thought

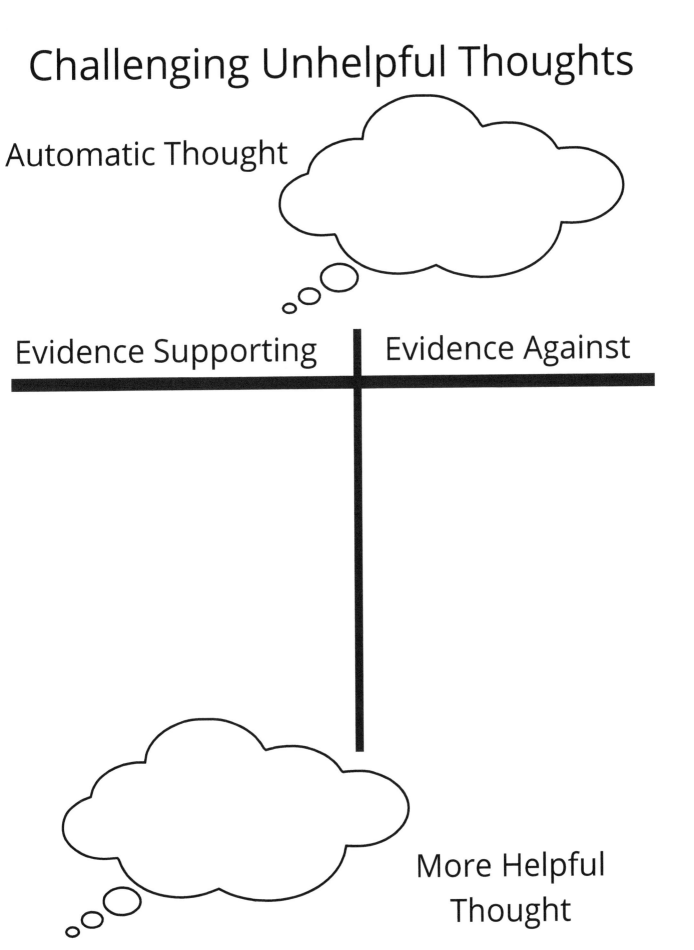

Evidence Supporting | Evidence Against

More Helpful
Thought

Alternative Thoughts

SITUATION	THOUGHTS	FEELINGS (RATE 0-10)	ALTERNATIVE THOUGHT	FEELINGS (RATE 0-10)
CGM alarm goes off in class.	Everyone will think I am weird and won't want to be my friend anymore.	Worried -7 Sad- 9	My alarm has gone off in class before and has never affected my friendships.	Worried-3 Sad-0

Let's bring down worry!
A little mathematics exercise!

A	Number of days _____ has had T1D...	_____
B	Number of lows _____ has had...	_____
C	Number of lows for which _____ has needed assistance...	_____
D	Number of lows for which _____ has needed assistance / total blood glucose checks _____ has done...	= ___ / ___ = ___%

What does all this mean?

These data show us that _____ VERY RARELY has a low when he needs assistance. We also know _____ has NEVER had a severe low where he needed glucagon. The chances that _____ will have a severe low are...VERY LOW.

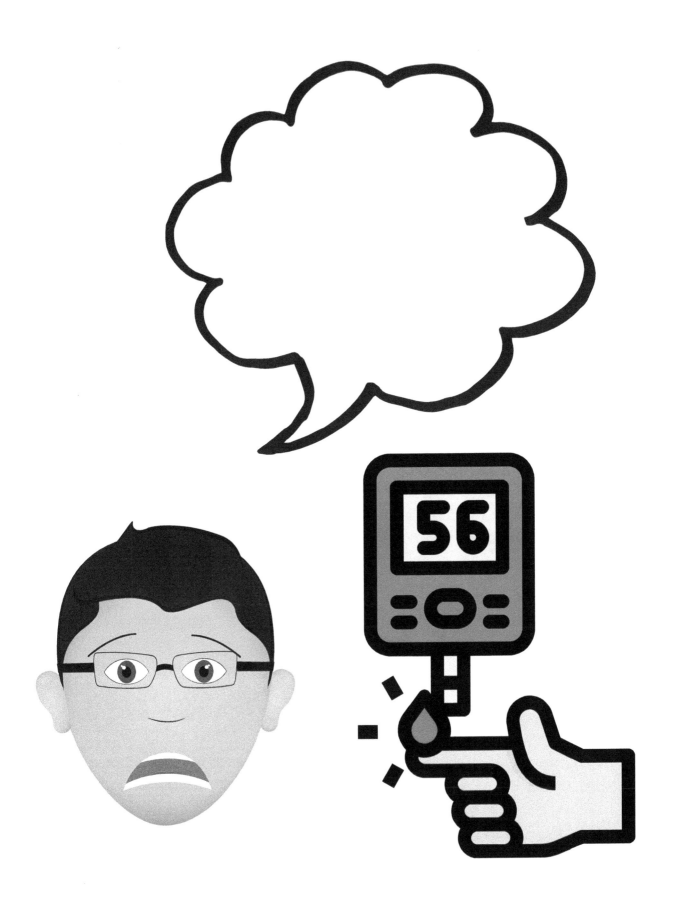

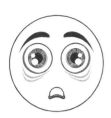

10

9

8

7

6

5

4

3

2

1

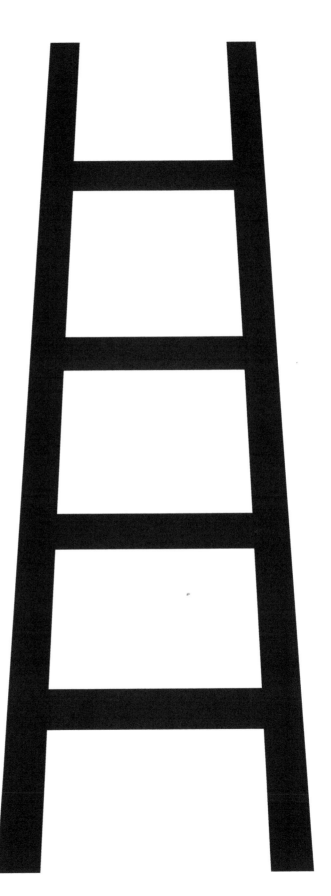

Phobia: Answering questions about T1D

Cut out the activities below and then work with your therapist or parent to place them on your fear ladder.

Tell therapist
what you know
about T1D

Tell friends
some facts
about T1D

Tell strangers
about T1D

Tell parents
about T1D

Tell stuffed
animals about
T1D

Think of unhelpful or
judgmental comments
others may make (like
"Did you eat too much
sugar?") and
practice answers

Think of questions others
may ask (like "How long
have you had T1D?") and
prepare answers

Practice answering
questions with adults who
work in your
therapist's office

Phobia: People finding out about T1D

Cut out the activities below and then work with your therapist or parent
to place them on your fear ladder.

Wear a t-shirt
about T1D
awareness

Teach someone
about T1D

Tell someone
you have T1D

Wear Medical ID
jewelry

Make eye
contact with
a person who
just learned you
have T1D

Stand in a public area
holding a sign that
states facts about T1D,
or "I have diabetes"

Stand nearby when
your parent tells
someone you have
T1D

Wear decorative
accents with your
devices (like colorful
adhesive or bag for
holding insulin pump)

Wear a T1D
device where
it's visible at
HOME

Wear a T1D
device where
it's visible at
SCHOOL

Wear a T1D
device where
it's visible in
PUBLIC

Phobia: Completing care tasks in front of others

Cut out the activities below and then work with your therapist or parent to place them on your fear ladder.

Show therapist your T1D devices and talk about them

Allow friend to watch you perform T1D tasks with school nurse

Show therapist how to use T1D devices

Bring a friend to school nurse with you

Complete T1D tasks in front of one or more friends

Complete T1D tasks in front of one or more family members

Complete T1D tasks with your parents nearby and then with them further away

Check blood glucose at a table in a restaurant –KEEP YOUR HAND UNDER THE TABLE

Check blood glucose at a table in a restaurant –KEEP YOUR HAND ABOVE THE TABLE

Complete T1D tasks in front of your therapist

Organize your T1D bag (meter, strips, low treatments, etc.) in front of someone else or in public

Phobia: Having high or low blood glucose symptoms in public

Cut out the activities below and then work with your therapist or parent
to place them on your fear ladder.

Pretend to trip
and fall in a
public setting

Pretend to walk
slower or in a
'wobbly' way as
if feeling weak

Take deep
breaths in a
busy area

Find a chair and
sit down in a
busy area

Put head
between knees
in public as
though feeling
dizzy or ill

Practice response to
"What's wrong with
you?"

Ask for space
in public

Find a chair and sit
down in the waiting
room of your clinic/
therapist's office

Sit on floor
in public

Take deep breaths
in the waiting room of
your clinic/therapist's
office

PRACTICING EXPOSURES

COGNITIVE COPING

Things I can say to myself/my brain:

PARENTS/CAREGIVERS

Things my parents/caregivers can do to support me:

People react differently to feared situations. Some people have a "flight or fight" response and others may feel weak and faint. Discuss with your therapist how you react when you are afraid.

KEEPING MY BODY CALM

"Fight or Flight." Strategies I can use to keep my "fight or flight" (blood pressure and heart rate increase) in control:

Weak and Faint. Muscle tension strategies I can use to keep my blood pressure and heart rate elevated:

EXPOSURES I AM WORKING ON

Fear Thermometer

10 the most scared and upset I have ever felt, I want to run away

9 very scared, thinking I can't do this, my fear is too much, panicking

8 very scared, wishing I could be somewhere else

7 scared, thinking something bad might happen

6 scared, uncomfortable, very tense

5 nervous, tense, worrying about what will happen

4 sort of nervous, feeling tense

3 a little worried and nervous

2 pretty easy, feeling a little bit nervous

1 easy, feeling good

0 very easy, feeling great, no anxiety

Chapter 8
Additional Considerations

To provide comprehensive care for youth with T1D, the mental health provider must consider the important effects of pain, sleep, and considerations related to siblings.

Pain

Research on pain in diabetes primarily focuses on adults with diabetes and the chronic pain that is associated with long-term complications (e.g., diabetic polyneuropathy or nerve pain caused by long-term hyperglycemia). Children and adolescents with T1D also experience general pain that affects their functioning.[162] Intermittent pain is reported during quarterly diabetes clinic visits in ~50% of adolescents with T1D, with the most common types reported being gastrointestinal and central nervous system pain, including stomach pain and migraines. These general pain symptoms are more typically found in girls and are related to increased hospital utilization and decreased physical activity.[162] Helping young people with T1D who experience interim general pain increase their physical activity on a daily basis is recommended.[162]

Young people with T1D also experience pain related to routine medical procedures and blood draws to screen for health concerns (e.g., cholesterol, thyroid function, celiac disease assessment). Borrowing from the literature on pain experiences with venipuncture laboratory draws and immunizations, recommendations include 1) teaching the child to engage in breathing exercises (e.g., party blower, bubbles, deep breaths); 2) child-directed distractions (e.g., music or a story playing in headphones, watching cartoons); 3) nurse-directed distractions (e.g., interacting using age-appropriate toys); and 4) cognitive behavioral interventions (e.g., combining breathing with positive self-statements).[163] Distraction and coaching from the parents are not generally successful.[164] In addition, some types of adult reassurances (e.g., making statements such as "Don't worry") during laboratory blood draws often paradoxically increase childrens' distress because these verbalizations signal the child about the adult's own fear and anxiety.[164] Uninformative reassurance (e.g., "It's okay") and informative reassurance (e.g., "It's almost done") were equally ineffective compared with distraction (e.g., "Look at the fish").[164] Reassurance by adults is a complex interaction that involves one's facial expression, vocal tone, and verbal content. It is recommended that for adults to help reduce distress and pain experiences in children and adolescents during laboratory draws, distraction strategies should be used, and that any adult verbal reassurance that occurs needs to be accompanied by a happy facial expression (instead of fearful) and a rising vocal tone (i.e., playful, silly).

One of the most common sources of diabetes-specific acute pain is injection pain, including from syringes, insulin pens, technology device insertion sets (insulin pumps and continuous glucose monitoring), blood glucose checks, and glucagon injections. If the pain associated with these T1D management tasks is not addressed adequately, young people with T1D may develop anxiety symptoms and avoid completing these self-management behaviors as a maladaptive coping technique. If children with T1D skip insulin doses, do not complete blood glucose checks as frequently as needed, or delay changing their technology devices as often as recommended, glycemic control will likely worsen across time.

There are evidence-based pharmacologic (e.g., numbing cream and vapocoolant spray) and nonpharmacologic (e.g., distraction, staying in a calm state, and feeling supported by adults) interventions that reduce pain associated with injections in children. Although the pharmacologic interventions decrease the experience of pain, these strategies are often cumbersome to complete repeatedly each day or use effectively in multiple types of environments.[165] Nonpharmacologic interventions are based on the gate control theory of pain,[166] which suggests that when pain signals from around the body travel to the brain, they have to pass through "gates" to be fully experienced by the individual. If the gates are closed (or partially closed), then the pain message from the body does not pass fully through the gates to the brain and therefore is not experienced as negatively. Therefore, recommendations for nonpharmacologic pain treatment focus on teaching individuals strategies to that can "close the gates." Calming strategies help individuals 1) stay out of the fight-or-flight mode, 2) distract themselves from their pain experience, and 3) stay in a positive emotional state during potentially painful tasks.[167]

Two examples of nonpharmacologic distraction devices that have been specifically shown to be effective in immediately reducing insulin injection pain in young people with T1D are Buzzy (a handheld cold application and vibration device placed directly on the skin just above the injection site) and ShotBlocker (a device that has a number of blunt contact points that saturate the sensory signals around the injection site).[159] The competing sensory input to the brain from these devices helps close the gates and reduce the pain experience from insulin injections. Both devices can be cleaned easily and used repeatedly, and are available for purchase without a prescription. ShotBlocker showed greater benefit than Buzzy in reducing pain reports from both children and independent observers.[165]

Sleep

Youth with T1D have shorter sleep duration than young people without T1D, which compromises self-management and glycemic outcomes.[168] Children <7 years of age who have T1D often do not meet recommended sleep recommendations and they experience more nighttime awakenings, higher blood glucoses, and increased glycemic variability on weekends when sleep routines are less predictable.[169] Only 20% of adolescents with T1D sleep the recommended number of hours per school night, and adolescents who do not sleep a sufficient amount are more likely to experience negative consequences the following day, such as feeling tired and irritable, falling asleep in school, having depressed mood, and drinking caffeinated beverages.[170] Circadian misalignment, or "social jet lag," also occurs during adolescence. Adolescents exhibit a later circadian phase than adults. In combination with early awakening during the school week, social jet lag may lead to the accumulation of sleep deficiency in adolescents with T1D.[171–173] Moreover, greater circadian misalignment is associated with increased insulin requirements.[174] Adolescents with sleep difficulties are also more likely to be diagnosed with a mood disorder and demonstrate lower problem-solving ability and greater avoidance of difficult tasks.[175] Those who spend less time in deep sleep have more episodes of hyperglycemia, greater behavioral difficulties, increased depressive symptoms, worse quality of life, and poorer school functioning.[176] In contrast, increased sleep duration is associated with an increase in completion of T1D self-management behaviors.[177] Nocturnal hypoglycemia and hyperglycemia may impair sleep and affect quality of life because they lead to more nighttime awakenings.[178] Given the high fear of hypoglycemia during the night among parents of children with T1D, there is a need to consider the effect of T1D on parents' sleep quality and quantity.[179]

For young people with clinically significant sleep concerns or in whom a medical etiology for a sleep disorder is suspected, referral to a primary care provider and sleep specialist may be warranted. However, many behavioral and T1D-specific sleep concerns can be effectively addressed using interventions to promote sleep hygiene and to reduce nighttime awakenings caused by diabetes-related factors. Sleep hygiene means having both a nighttime sleep environment and daytime routine that promotes consistent, uninterrupted sleep. Mental health professionals can consult with diabetes care providers to ensure overnight T1D management needs are met in a way that minimally conflicts with sleep hygiene recommendations. For example, diabetes care providers can advise about the need for overnight glucose checks and may provide guidance about changing overnight glucose target ranges on a continuous glucose monitor to minimize unnecessary audio alerts.

Supporting Siblings of Youth with T1D

Even when only one child in a family has T1D, it is often considered a condition that affects the whole family.[181] As detailed in previous sections, parents of children with T1D often take the most responsibility for ensuring T1D management tasks are completed and they are at elevated risk for experiencing diabetes distress and other mood or anxiety symptoms.[57] Most research focused on other family members involves parents, and there is a significant gap in the literature on siblings of children who have T1D.[181] However, siblings can have a wide array of experiences related to their sibling's T1D and its management demands.[182]

Siblings often perceive a shift in parents' attention toward the child with a health condition.[183] Research with families of young people with T1D suggests that siblings in this population may experience jealousy regarding this change in the family dynamic, as well as frustration with how demands related to T1D may affect family activities.[181,182] For example, T1D management tasks (e.g., treating a low glucose) may delay or prevent family activities, or T1D needs may dominate the conversation or focus of activities (e.g., managing blood glucose around meals). Across health conditions, siblings report high degrees of concern about a sibling with a health condition, and some siblings experience mood concerns, although a common theme is siblings being reluctant to disclose their distress in order to reduce burden on their parents.[182,183]

There are positive aspects of having a sibling with T1D or another health condition. Some siblings perceive an increase in family closeness and support of one another,[183] including between the siblings with and without T1D.[182] In some cases, siblings become involved in disease management tasks to support their family and help their sibling with the health condition.[183] Most of this research was conducted in other health conditions, but similar patterns may be observed in families of children with T1D.[184,185]

Supporting families of youth with T1D may benefit from assessing whether there are siblings, what their experiences are with their sibling's diabetes, and to what degree and how the family system addresses the needs of siblings without diabetes. Depending on the role of the mental health professional (e.g., family therapy versus individual diabetes-related consultation) and the siblings' ages, amount of distress, and experiences, the degree of direct support for siblings may vary. If parents are concerned about siblings' well-being, possible strategies may include the following:

1. Discussing ways for the parents and family to support the individual needs of the sibling unrelated to T1D could include working to have regular opportunities for "special" time for the parent and each sibling in which T1D is not a focus and the sibling without diabetes chooses the activity. If siblings have symptoms of mood, anxiety, or other psychosocial or cognitive concerns, a referral for their own assessment and treatment may be warranted.

2. Addressing concerns siblings have about T1D or the health and safety of their sibling with T1D by providing age-appropriate basic education about T1D may help alleviate siblings' worries. Encouraging parents to teach siblings to identify signs of urgent diabetes-related problems (e.g., symptoms of low blood glucose) can give siblings the tools to know when their sibling with T1D needs immediate help. However, their capacity to use this information should be assessed based on age, developmental stage, and other individual factors. Collaborating with the child's pediatric diabetes care team (especially diabetes educators) can be a good way to ensure siblings have access to educational materials that are appropriate for their age and learning level.

3. Finding opportunities to engage in positive experiences related to T1D will help siblings support their sibling with T1D. Even young children may be able to help with T1D management tasks, such as fetching supplies or distracting the child with T1D during unpleasant activities (e.g., changing insertion sites for diabetes devices). Recognizing when siblings are being helpful and praising them can make them feel appreciated and helpful. Some siblings may be interested in getting involved in T1D activities on a broader level, such as teaching their classmates about T1D or attending diabetes-related community events, fundraising activities, or diabetes camps. It is important for these activities to be optional for siblings without T1D; pressuring them to engage with T1D-related activities may backfire if they do not want to participate.

Chapter 8 Worksheets

Getting a Good Night's Sleep with T1D

Technology

Avoid screen time 1 hour before bed. Light triggers body to stay awake.

Bedroom

Quiet and dark (except for night light)!

Bed is for sleeping only!

Routine

Try to go to bed at the same time every night.

Keep weekday and weekend wake times within 1 hour.

Create and follow a relaxing bedtime routine.

T1D Sleep

Do I have snacks or juice to treat a low?

If using phone for T1D management, try turning off other apps on phone (i.e., text messaging).

Duration

Preschoolers: 10-13 hrs.
School age: 9-11 hrs.
Teenagers: 8-10 hrs.

My bedtime is _____,
and I get up at _____.

Resources

National and International Professional Diabetes Organizations and Websites

American Diabetes Association (www.diabetes.org)
- Mental health provider directory listing: https://professional.diabetes.org/mhp_listing
- Diabetes Education 101 for the Behavioral Health Provider Program (video on-demand, psychology continuing education credits available): https://professional.diabetes.org/meetings/mental-health-provider-diabetes-education-video-demand-program
- *Diabetes and Emotional Health: A Practical Guide for Health Professionals Supporting Adults with Type 1 and Type 2 Diabetes* (free e-book published by the American Diabetes Association): https://professional.diabetes.org/meetings/mentalhealthworkbook
- Mental health information: www.diabetes.org/healthy-living/mental-health
- Safe at School state laws: www.diabetes.org/tools-support/know-your-rights/safe-at-school-state-laws

Association of Diabetes Care & Education Specialists (www.diabeteseducator.org)
- Language use guidelines: www.diabeteseducator.org/practice/practice-tools/app-resources/diabetes-language-paper

Behavioral Diabetes Institute (https://behavioraldiabetes.org/resources)
- Resources and videos for health care professionals: https://behavioraldiabetes.org/programs/health-care-professionals
- Assessment scales and measures: https://behavioraldiabetes.org/scales-and-measures

Close Concerns (www.closeconcerns.com)

Diabetes Wise: www.pro.diabeteswise.org

International Society for Pediatric and Adolescent Diabetes (www.ispad.org)

JDRF (www.jdrf.org)
- Resources for health care professionals: www.jdrf.org/t1d-resources/hcp

National Institute of Diabetes and Digestive and Kidney Diseases (www.niddk.nih.gov)
- *Diabetes in America, 3rd ed.:* www.niddk.nih.gov/about-niddk/strategic-plans-reports/diabetes-in-america-3rd-edition

Books for Professionals

American Diabetes Association. Diabetes books. Arlington, VA, American Diabetes Association. Available from https://shopdiabetes.org/collections/professional-books

Anderson BJ, Rubin RR. *Practical Psychology for Diabetes Clinicians: Effective Techniques for Key Behavioral Issues.* 2nd ed. Arlington, VA, American Diabetes Association, 2003

Anderson BJ, Wolpert HA, Harris MA. *Transitions in Care: Meeting the Challenges of Type 1 Diabetes in Young Adults.* Arlington, VA, American Diabetes Association, 2009

Delamater AM, Marrero D. *Behavioral Diabetes: Social Ecological Perspectives for Pediatric and Adult Populations.* New York, Springer, 2020

Harris MA, Hood KK, Weissberg-Benchell J. *Teens with Diabetes: A Clinician's Guide.* Arlington, VA, American Diabetes Association, 2014

Nezu AM, Nezu CM, D'Zurilla T. *Problem-Solving Therapy: A Treatment Manual.* New York, Springer, 2013

Peters AL, Laffel LM. *American Diabetes Association/JDRF Type 1 Diabetes Sourcebook.* Arlington, VA, American Diabetes Association, 2013

Robin AL, Foster SL. *Negotiating Parent–Adolescent Conflict: A Behavioral–Family Systems Approach.* New York, Guilford Press, 1989

Tamborlane WV. *Diabetes in Children and Adolescents: A Guide to Diagnosis and Management.* Totowa, NJ, Humana Press, 2021

Young-Hyman D. *Psychosocial Care for People With Diabetes.* Arlington, VA, American Diabetes Association, 2013

Books for People with Diabetes

Brown A. *Bright Spots & Landmines: The Diabetes Guide I Wish Someone Had Handed Me.* San Francisco, diaTribe Foundation, 2017

Hatchell S. *Shia Learns About Insulin.* New York, JDRF, 2020

Hood KK. *Type 1 Teens: A Guide to Managing Your Life with Diabetes.* Washington, DC, Magination Press, 2010

McCarthy M. *Raising Teens with Diabetes: A Survival Guide for Parents.* Ann Arbor, Spry Publishing, 2013

Polonsky WH. *Diabetes Burnout: What to Do When You Can't Take It Anymore.* Arlington, VA, American Diabetes Association, 1999

Scheiner G. *Think Like a Pancreas.* 3rd ed. New York, Hachette, 2020

Simms S. *The World's Worst Diabetes Mom: Real-Life Stories of Parenting a Child with Type 1 Diabetes.* Pittsburgh, Spark, 2019

Wysocki T. *The Ten Keys to Helping Your Child Grow Up with Diabetes.* 2nd ed. Arlington, VA, American Diabetes Association, 2003

Diabetes Organizations and Websites for the Diabetes Community

American Diabetes Association Support Community: https://community.diabetes.org/home

Beyond Type 1: beyondtype1.org

Beyond Type 2: beyondtype2.org

Children with Diabetes: childrenwithdiabetes.com

Defeat Diabetes Foundation: https://defeatdiabetes.org/get-healthy/diabetes-support-groups/page/2

Diabetemoji Stickers: www.healthdesignby.us/diabetemoji

Diabetes Online Community: www.diabeteseducator.org/living-with-diabetes/peer-support

Diabetes Mine: www.healthline.com/diabetesmine

Diabetes Sisters: www.diabetessisters.org

Diabetes Wise: www.diabeteswise.org

diaTribe Learn: Making Sense of Diabetes: www.diatribe.org

Diversity in Diabetes: www.diversityindiabetes.org

JDRF Community: www.jdrf.org/community

JDRF Teen Toolkit: www.jdrf.org/wp-content/uploads/2013/10/JDRFTEENTOOLKIT.pdf

T1 Everyday Magic: www.t1everydaymagic.com

The Diabetes Link (https://www.thediabeteslink.org)

References

1. American Diabetes Association. Glycemic Targets: Standards of Care in Diabetes-2023. *Diabetes Care* 2023;46(Suppl. 1):S97-S110

2. Nurmi JE. Thinking about and acting upon the future: development of future orientation across the life span. In: Strathman A, Joireman J, eds. *Understanding Behavior in the Context of Time: Theory, Research, and Application*. Mahwah, NJ, Lawrence Erlbaum Associates, 2005, p. 31–57

3. Foster NC, Beck RW, Miller KM, et al. State of type 1 diabetes management and outcomes from the T1D exchange in 2016-2018. *Diabetes Technol Ther* 2019;21:66–72

4. Rausch JR, Hood KK, Delamater A, et al. Changes in treatment adherence and glycemic control during the transition to adolescence in type 1 diabetes. *Diabetes Care* 2012;35:1219–1224

5. Miller KM, Beck RW, Bergenstal RM, et al. Evidence of a strong association between frequency of self-monitoring of blood glucose and hemoglobin A1c levels in T1D exchange clinic registry participants. *Diabetes Care* 2013;36:2009–2014

6. Kichler JC, Harris MA, Weissberg-Benchell J. Contemporary roles of the pediatric psychologist in diabetes care. *Curr Diabetes Rev* 2015;11:210–221

7. Agiostratidou G, Anhalt H, Ball D, et al. Standardizing clinically meaningful outcome measures beyond HbA1c for type 1 diabetes: a consensus report of the American Association of Clinical Endocrinologists, the American Association of Diabetes Educators, the American Diabetes Association, the Endocrine Society, JDRF International, The Leona M. and Harry B. Helmsley Charitable Trust, the Pediatric Endocrine Society, and the T1D Exchange. *Diabetes Care* 2017;40:1622–1630

8. American Diabetes Association. Facilitating Positive Health Behaviors and Well-being to Improve Health Outcomes: Standards of Care in Diabetes-2023. *Diabetes Care* 2023;46(Suppl. 1):S97-S110

9. Kahkoska AR, Shay CM, Crandell J, et al. Association of race and ethnicity with glycemic control and hemoglobin A1c levels in youth with type 1 diabetes. *JAMA Netw Open* 2018;1:e181851

10. Children and Adolescents: Standards of Care in Diabetes-2023. *Diabetes Care* 2023;46 (Suppl. 1):S230-S253

11. Sparling KM. *Rage Bolus & Other Poems*. Kerri Sparling, 2018

12. Gallagher KAS, DeSalvo D, Gregory J, Hilliard ME. Medical and psychological considerations for carbohydrate-restricted diets in youth with type 1 diabetes. *Curr Diab Rep* 2019;19:27

13. Miller KM, Foster NC, Beck RW, et al. Current state of type 1 diabetes treatment in the U.S.: updated data from the T1D Exchange clinic registry. *Diabetes Care* 2015;38:971–978

14. Sullivan-Bolyai S, Deatrick J, Gruppuso P, et al. Constant vigilance: mothers' work parenting young children with type 1 diabetes. *J Pediatr Nurs* 2003;18:21–29

15. Litchman ML, Oser TK, Wawrzynski SE, et al. The underground exchange of diabetes medications and supplies: donating, trading, and borrowing, oh my! *J Diabetes Sci Technol* 2020;14:1000–1009

16. Eshtehardi SS, Anderson BJ, Cao VT, et al. On the money: parental perspectives about finances and type 1 diabetes in youth. *Clin Pract Pediatr Psychol* 2021;9:340–350

17. Herkert D, Vijayakumar P, Luo J, et al. Cost-related insulin underuse among patients with diabetes. *JAMA Intern Med* 2019;179:112–114

18. Blanchette JE, Toly VB, Wood JR. Financial stress in emerging adults with type 1 diabetes in the United States. *Pediatr Diabetes* 2021;22:807–815

19. Willner S, Whittemore R, Keene D. "Life or death": experiences of insulin insecurity among adults with type 1 diabetes in the United States. *SSM Popul Health* 2020;11:100624

20. American Diabetes Association. Diabetes technology: *Standards of Medical Care in Diabetes* 2021. *Diabetes Care* 2021;44:S85–S99

21. Prahalad P, Tanenbaum M, Hood K, Maahs DM. Diabetes technology: improving care, improving patient-reported outcomes and preventing complications in young people with type 1 diabetes. *Diabet Med* 2018;35:419–429

22. Sinisterra M, Hamburger S, Tully C, et al. Young children with type 1 diabetes: sleep, health-related quality of life, and continuous glucose monitor use. *Diabetes Technol Ther* 2020;22:639–642

23. Rosner B, Roman-Urrestarazu A. Health-related quality of life in paediatric patients with Type 1 diabetes mellitus using insulin infusion systems: a systematic review and meta-analysis. *PLoS One* 2019;14:e0217655

24. Messer LH, Tanenbaum M, Cook PF, et al. Cost, hassle, and on-body experience: barriers to diabetes device use in adolescents and potential intervention targets. *Diabetes Technol Ther* 2020;22:760–767

25. Hilliard ME, Levy W, Anderson BJ, et al. Benefits and barriers of continuous glucose monitoring in young children with type 1 diabetes. *Diabetes Technol Ther* 2019;21:493–498

26. Lai CW, Lipman T, Willi SM, Hawkes CP. Early racial/ethnic disparities in continuous glucose monitor use in pediatric type 1 diabetes. *Diabetes Technol Ther* 2021;23:763–767

27. Agarwal S, Schechter C, Gonzalez J, Long JA. Racial-ethnic disparities in diabetes technology use among young adults with type 1 diabetes. *Diabetes Technol Ther* 2021;23:306–313

28. Addala A, Auzanneau M, Miller K, et al. A decade of disparities in diabetes technology use and HbA1c in pediatric type 1 diabetes: a transatlantic comparison. *Diabetes Care* 2021;44:133–140

29. Agarwal S, Crespo-Ramos G, Long JA, Miller VA. "I didn't really have a choice": qualitative analysis of racial-ethnic disparities in diabetes technology use among young adults with type 1 diabetes. *Diabetes Technol Ther* 2021;23

30. Addala A, Hanes S, Naranjo D, et al. Provider implicit bias impacts pediatric type 1 diabetes technology recommendations in the United States: findings from the Gatekeeper Study. *J Diabetes Sci Technol* 2021;15:1027–1033

31. Hunter CM. Understanding diabetes and the role of psychology in its prevention and treatment. *Am Psychol* 2016;71:515–525

32. Hagger V, Hendrieckx C, Sturt J, et al. Diabetes distress among adolescents with type 1 diabetes: a systematic review. *Curr Diab Rep* 2016;16:9

33. Nieuwesteeg A, Pouwer F, van der Kamp R, et al. Quality of life of children with type 1 diabetes: a systematic review. *Curr Diabetes Rev* 2012;8:434–443

34. Naranjo D, Mulvaney S, McGrath M, et al. Predictors of self-management in pediatric type 1 diabetes: individual, family, systemic, and technologic influences. *Curr Diab Rep* 2014;14:544

35. Markowitz JT, Garvey KC, Laffel LM. Developmental changes in the roles of patients and families in type 1 diabetes management. *Curr Diabetes Rev* 2015;11:231–238

36. Young MT, Lord JH, Patel NJ, et al. Good cop, bad cop: quality of parental involvement in type 1 diabetes management in youth. *Curr Diab Rep* 2014;14:546

37. Hilliard ME, Powell PW, Anderson BJ. Evidence-based behavioral interventions to promote diabetes management in children, adolescents, and families. *Am Psychol* 2016;71:590–601

38. Young-Hyman D, de Groot M, Hill-Briggs F, et al. Psychosocial care for people with diabetes: a position statement of the American Diabetes Association. *Diabetes Care* 2016;39:2126–2140

39. Delamater AM, de Wit M, McDarby V, et al. ISPAD clinical practice consensus guidelines 2018: psychological care of children and adolescents with type 1 diabetes. *Pediatr Diabetes* 2018;19(Suppl. 27):237–249

40. Vogel ME, Kanzler KE, Aikens JE, Goodie JL. Integration of behavioral health and primary care: current knowledge and future directions. *J Behav Med* 2017;40:69–84

41. de Wit M, Pulgaron ER, Pattino-Fernandez AM, Delamater AM. Psychological support for children with diabetes: are the guidelines being met? *J Clin Psychol Med Settings* 2014;21:190–199

42. Gray WN, Monaghan MC, Gilleland Marchak J, et al. Psychologists and the transition from pediatrics to adult health care. *J Adolesc Health* 2015;57:468–474

43. Barry-Menkhaus SA, Wagner DV, Riley AR. Small interventions for big change: brief strategies for distress and self-management amongst youth with type 1 diabetes. *Curr Diab Rep* 2020;20:3

44. Hill-Briggs F, Adler NE, Berkowitz SA, et al. Social determinants of health and diabetes: a scientific review. *Diabetes Care* 2020;44:258–279

45. Streisand R, Monaghan M. Young children with type 1 diabetes: challenges, research, and future directions. *Curr Diab Rep* 2014;14:520

46. Chiang JL, Maahs DM, Garvey KC, et al. Type 1 diabetes in children and adolescents: a position statement by the American Diabetes Association. *Diabetes Care* 2018;41:2026–2044

47. Monaghan M, Helgeson V, Wiebe D. Type 1 diabetes in young adulthood. *Curr Diabetes Rev* 2015;11:239–250

48. Dickinson JK, Guzman SJ, Maryniuk MD, et al. The use of language in diabetes care and education. *Diabetes Care* 2017;40:1790–1799

49. Dickinson JK. The Experience of Diabetes-Related Language in Diabetes Care. *Diabetes Spectr*. 2018 Feb;31(1):58-64. doi: 10.2337/ds16-0082. PMID: 29456427; PMCID: PMC5813309.

50. Linguistic Society of America. Guidelines for inclusive language. Available from: https://www.linguisticsociety.org/resource/guidelines-inclusive-language

51. Bowes S, Lowes L, Warner J, Gregory JW. Chronic sorrow in parents of children with type 1 diabetes. *J Adv Nurs* 2009;65:992–1000

52. Whittemore R, Jaser S, Chao A, et al. Psychological experience of parents of children with type 1 diabetes: a systematic mixed-studies review. *Diabetes Educ* 2012;38:562–579

53. Yi-Frazier JP, Cochrane K, Whitlock K, et al. Trajectories of acute diabetes-specific stress in adolescents with type 1 diabetes and their caregivers within the first year of diagnosis. *J Pediatr Psychol* 2018;43:645–653

54. Grey M; Coping Skills Training for Youths With Diabetes. *Diabetes Spectr* 1 May 2011; 24 (2): 70–75. https://doi.org/10.2337/diaspect.24.2.70

55. Wu Y, Zhang YY, Zhang YT, et al. Effectiveness of resilience-promoting interventions in adolescents with diabetes mellitus: a systematic review and meta-analysis. *World J Pediatr.* 2023 Apr;19(4):323-339. doi:10.1007/s12519-022-00666-7. Epub 2022 Dec 19. PMID: 36534296; PMCID: PMC9761642.

56. Jaser SS. Family interaction in pediatric diabetes. *Curr Diab Rep* 2011;11:480–485

57. Helgeson VS, Reynolds KA, Siminerio L, et al. Parent and adolescent distribution of responsibility for diabetes self-care: links to health outcomes. *J Pediatr Psychol* 2008;33:497–508

58. Ingerski LM, Anderson BJ, Dolan LM, Hood KK. Blood glucose monitoring and glycemic control in adolescence: contribution of diabetes-specific responsibility and family conflict. *J Adolesc Health* 2010;47:191–197

59. Kelly CS, Berg CA, Ramsey MA, et al. Relationships and the development of transition readiness skills into early emerging adulthood for individuals with type 1 diabetes. *Child Health Care* 2018;47:308–325

60. Butler AM, Hilliard ME, Titus C, Rodriguez E, Al-Gadi I, Cole-Lewis Y, et al. Barriers and Facilitators to Involvement in Children's Diabetes Management Among Minority Parents. *J Pediatr Psychol.* 2020;45(8):946-56

61. Hsin O, La Greca AM, Valenzuela J, Moine CT, Delamater A. Adherence and glycemic control among Hispanic youth with type 1 diabetes: role of family involvement and acculturation. J Pediatr Psychol. 2010;35(2):156-66

62. Palladino DK, Helgeson VS. Friends or foes? A review of peer influence on self-care and glycemic control in adolescents with type 1 diabetes. *J Pediatr Psychol* 2012;37:591–603

63. Walker AF, Schatz DA, Johnson C, Silverstein JH, Rohrs HJ. Disparities in social support systems for youths with type 1 diabetes. Clin Diabetes. 2015;33(2):62-9

64. Weissberg-Benchell J, Rychlik K. Diabetes camp matters: assessing families' views of their diabetes camp experience. *Pediatr Diabetes* 2017;18:853–860

65. Valenzuela JM, Martin MT, Records S, O"Neal K, Mueller K, Wolf RM. Racial ethnic disparities in diabetes youth participating in diabetes summer camps. Diabetes. 2018;67 (S1)

66. Wiebe DJ, Berg CA, Mello D, Kelly CS. Self- and social regulation in type 1 diabetes management during late adolescence and emerging adulthood. *Curr Diab Rep* 2018;18:23

67. Fiese BH. Routines and rituals: opportunities for participation in family health. *OTJR Occup Particip Health* 2007;27(Suppl. 1):41S–49S

68. Verplanken B. By force of habit. In: Steptoe A, ed. *Handbook of Behavioral Medicine*. New York, Springer, 2010

69. Herge WM, Streisand R, Chen R, et al. Family and youth factors associated with health beliefs and health outcomes in youth with type 1 diabetes. *J Pediatr Psychol* 2012;37:980–989

70. Pierce JS, Jordan SS, Arnau RC. Development and validation of the pediatric diabetes routines questionnaire for adolescents. *J Clin Psychol Med Settings* 2019;26:47–58

71. Pyatak E. Participation in occupation and diabetes self-management in emerging adulthood. *Am J Occup Ther* 2011;65:462–469

72. Greening L, Stoppelbein L, Konishi C, et al. Child routines and youths' adherence to treatment for type 1 diabetes. *J Pediatr Psychol* 2007;32:437–447

73. Butler AM, Hilliard ME, Titus C, Rodriguez E, Al-Gadi I, Cole-Lewis Y, et al. Barriers and facilitators to involvement in children's diabetes management among minority parents. *J Pediatr Psychol.* 2020;45(8):946-56

74. Hanna KM, Hansen JR. Habits and routines during transitions among emerging adults with type 1 diabetes. *West J Nurs Res* 2020;42:446–453

75. Spagnola M, Fiese B. Family Routines and Rituals: A Context for Development in the Lives of Young Children. *Infants & Young Children* Vol. 20, No. 4, pp. 284–299. 2007. Wolters Kluwer Health | Lippincott Williams & Wilkins.

76. Maranda L, Lau M, Stewart SM, Gupta OT. A novel behavioral intervention in adolescents with type 1 diabetes mellitus improves glycemic control: preliminary results from a pilot randomized control trial. *Diabetes Educ* 2015;41:224–230

77. Redondo MJ, Callender CS, Gonynor C, et al. Diabetes care provider perceptions on family challenges of pediatric type 1 diabetes. *Diabetes Res Clin Pract* 2017;129:203–205

78. Drotar D, Ittenbach R, Rohan JM, et al. Diabetes management and glycemic control in youth with type 1 diabetes: test of a predictive model. *J Behav Med* 2013;36:234–245

79. Rybak TM, Ali JS, Berlin KS, et al. Patterns of family functioning and diabetes-specific conflict in relation to glycemic control and health-related quality of life among youth with type 1 diabetes. *J Pediatr Psychol* 2017;42:40–51

80. Savin KL, Hamburger ER, Monzon AD, et al. Diabetes-specific family conflict: informant discrepancies and the impact of parental factors. *J Fam Psychol* 2018;32:157–163

81. Anderson BJ, Coyne JC. "Miscarried helping" in the families of children and adolescents with chronic diseases. In: Johnson JH, Johnson SB, eds. *Advances in Child Health Psychology*. Gainesville, FL, University of Florida Press, 1991, p. 167–177

82. Weinger K, O'Donnell KA, Ritholz MD. Adolescent views of diabetes-related parent conflict and support: a focus group analysis. *J Adolesc Health.* 2001 Nov;29(5):330-6. doi: 10.1016/s1054-139x(01)00270-1. PMID: 11691594; PMCID: PMC1592605.

83. Campbell MS, Wang J, Cheng Y, et al. Diabetes-specific family conflict and responsibility among emerging adults with type 1 diabetes. *J Fam Psychol* 2019;33:788–796

84. Anderson BJ, Brackett J, Ho J, Laffel LMB. An intervention to promote family teamwork in diabetes management tasks: relationships among parental involvement, adherence to blood glucose monitoring, and glycemic control in young adolescents with type 1 diabetes. Mahwah, NJ, Lawrence Erlbaum Associates, 2000

85. Wysocki T, Harris MA, Greco P, et al. Randomized, controlled trial of behavior therapy for families of adolescents with insulin-dependent diabetes mellitus. *J Pediatr Psychol* 2000;25:23–33

86. Wysocki T, Iannotti R, Weissberg-Benchell J, et al. Diabetes problem solving by youths with type 1 diabetes and their caregivers: measurement, validation, and longitudinal associations with glycemic control. *J Pediatr Psychol* 2008;33:875–884

87. Wysocki T, Harris MA, Buckloh LM, et al. Effects of behavioral family systems therapy for diabetes on adolescents' family relationships, treatment adherence, and metabolic control. *J Pediatr Psychol* 2006;31:928–938

88. Hilliard ME, Eshtehardi SS, Minard CG, et al. Strengths-based, clinic integrated nonrandomized pilot intervention to promote type 1 diabetes adherence and well being. *J Pediatr Psychol* 2019;44:5–15

89. Hilliard ME, Cao VT, Eshtehardi SS, et al. Type 1 doing well: pilot feasibility and acceptability study of a strengths-based mHealth app for parents of adolescents with type 1 diabetes. *Diabetes Technol Ther* 2020;22:835–845

90. Messer LH, Johnson R, Driscoll KA, Jones J. Best friend or spy: a qualitative metasynthesis on the impact of continuous glucose monitoring on life with Type 1 diabetes. *Diabet Med* 2018;35:409–418

91. Rose M, Aronow L, Breen S, Tully C, Hilliard ME, Butler AM, et al. Considering culture: a review of pediatric behavioral intervention research in type 1 diabetes. *Curr Diab Rep.* 2018;18(4):16

92: Forlenza GP, Messer LH, Berget C, Wadwa RP, Driscoll KA. Biopsychosocial factors associated with satisfaction and sustained use of artificial pancreas technology and its components: a call to the technology field. *Curr Diab Rep.* 2018 Sep 26;18(11):114. doi: 10.1007/s11892-018-1078-1. PMID: 30259309; PMCID: PMC6535227.

93. Howe CJ, Morone J, Hawkes CP, Lipman TH. Racial disparities in technology use in children with type 1 diabetes: a qualitative content analysis of parents' perspectives. *Sci Diabetes Self Manag Care.* 2023 Feb;49(1):55-64. doi: 10.1177/26350106221145323. Epub 2023 Jan 6. PMID: 36609201.

94 Liu NF, Brown AS, Folias AE, et al. Stigma in people with type 1 or type 2 diabetes. *Clin Diabetes* 2017;35:27–34

95. Abdoli S, Hessler D, Vora A, et al. Experiences of diabetes burnout: a qualitative study among people with type 1 diabetes. *Am J Nurs* 2019;119:22–31

96. Lewis LF, Brower PM, Narkewicz S. "We operate as an organ": parent experiences of having a child with yype 1 diabetes in a rural area. *Sci Diabetes Self Manag Care.* 2023 Feb;49(1):35-45. doi: 10.1177/26350106221144962. Epub 2023 Jan 3. PMID: 36594452.

97. Buchberger B, Huppertz H, Krabbe L, et al. Symptoms of depression and anxiety in youth with type 1 diabetes: a systematic review and meta-analysis. *Psychoneuroendocrinology* 2016;70:70–84

98. Liu S, Leone M, Ludvigsson JF, et al. Association and familial coaggregation of childhood-onset type 1 diabetes with depression, anxiety, and stress-related disorders: a population-based cohort study. *Diabetes Care.* 2022 Sep 1;45(9):1987-1993. doi: 10.2337/dc21-1347. PMID: 35913075; PMCID: PMC9472496.

99. Hilliard ME, Wu YP, Rausch J, et al. Predictors of deteriorations in diabetes management and control in adolescents with type 1 diabetes. *J Adolesc Health* 2013;52:28–34

100. Berg CA, Wiebe DJ, Suchy Y, et al. Individual differences and day-to-day fluctuations in perceived self-regulation associated with daily adherence in late adolescents with type 1 diabetes. *J Pediatr Psychol* 2014;39:1038–1048

101. Vaid E, Lansing AH, Stanger C. Problems with self-regulation, family conflict, and glycemic control in adolescents experiencing challenges with managing type 1 diabetes. *J Pediatr Psychol* 2018;43: 525–533

102. Inverso H, LeStourgeon LM, Parmar A, et al. Demographic and glycemic factors linked with diabetes distress in teens with type 1 diabetes. *J Pediatr Psychol.* 2022 Sep 15;47(9):1081-1089. doi: 10.1093/jpepsy/jsac049. PMID: 35656859; PMCID: PMC9801711

103. Berlin KS, Hains AA, Kamody RC, Kichler JC, Davies WH. Differentiating peer and friend social information-processing effects on stress and glycemic control among youth with type 1 diabetes. J Pediatr Psychol. 2015 Jun;40(5):492-9. doi: 10.1093/jpepsy/jsu111. Epub 2015 Jan 18. PMID: 25602022.

104. Valenzuela JM, Records SE, Mueller KA, Martin MT, Wolf RM. Racial ethnic disparities in youth with type 1 diabetes participating in diabetes summer camps. *Diabetes Care.* 2020 Apr;43(4):903-905. doi: 10.2337/dc19-1502. Epub 2020 Jan 23. PMID: 31974104.

105. Pallayova M, Taheri S. Targeting diabetes distress: the missing piece of the successful type 1 diabetes management puzzle. *Diabetes Spectr.* 2014 May;27(2):143-9. doi: 10.2337/diaspect.27.2.143. PMID: 26246771; PMCID: PMC4522882.

106. Akbarizadeh M, Naderi Far M, Ghaljaei F. Prevalence of depression and anxiety among children with type 1 and type 2 diabetes: a systematic review and meta-analysis. *World J Pediatr.* 2022 Jan;18(1):16-26. doi: 10.1007/s12519-021-00485-2. Epub 2021 Nov 22. PMID: 34807367.

107. Musselman DL, Betan E, Larsen H, Phillips LS. Relationship of depression to diabetes types 1 and 2: epidemiology, biology, and treatment. *Biol Psychiatry* 2003;54:317–329

108. Hood KK, Lawrence JM, Anderson A, et al. Metabolic and inflammatory links to depression in youth with diabetes. *Diabetes Care* 2012;35:2443–2446

109. Mulvaney SA, Mara CA, Kichler JC, et al. A retrospective multisite examination of depression screening practices, scores, and correlates in pediatric diabetes care. *Transl Behav Med* 2021;11:122–131

110. Hood KK, Rausch JR, Dolan LM. Depressive symptoms predict change in glycemic control in adolescents with type 1 diabetes: rates, magnitude, and moderators of change. *Pediatr Diabetes* 2011;12:718–723

111. de Wit M, Snoek FJ. Depressive symptoms and unmet psychological needs of Dutch youth with type 1 diabetes: results of a web-survey. *Pediatr Diabetes* 2011;12:172–176

112. Herzer M, Vesco A, Ingerski LM, et al. Explaining the family conflict–glycemic control link through psychological variables in adolescents with type 1 diabetes. *J Behav Med* 2011;34:268–274

113. Hilliard ME, Herzer M, Dolan LM, Hood KK. Psychological screening in adolescents with type 1 diabetes predicts outcomes one year later. *Diabetes Res Clin Pract* 2011;94:39–44

114. McGrady ME, Hood KK. Depressive symptoms in adolescents with type 1 diabetes: associations with longitudinal outcomes. *Diabetes Res Clin Pract* 2010;88:e35–e37

115. Guo J, Whittemore R, Grey M, et al. Diabetes self-management, depressive symptoms, quality of life and metabolic control in youth with type 1 diabetes in China. *J Clin Nurs* 2013;22:69–79

116. Baucom KJ, Queen TL, Wiebe DJ, et al. Depressive symptoms, daily stress, and adherence in late adolescents with type 1 diabetes. *Health Psychol* 2015;34:522–530

117. McGrady ME, Laffel L, Drotar D, et al. Depressive symptoms and glycemic control in adolescents with type 1 diabetes: mediational role of blood glucose monitoring. *Diabetes Care* 2009;32:804–806

118. Polonsky WH, Fisher L, Earles J, et al. Assessing psychosocial distress in diabetes: development of the diabetes distress scale. *Diabetes Care* 2005;28:626–631

119. Abdoli S, Hessler D, Vora A, et al. Descriptions of diabetes burnout from individuals with type 1 diabetes: an analysis of YouTube videos. *Diabet Med* 2020;37:1344–1351

120. Fisher L, Polonsky WH, Hessler D. Addressing diabetes distress in clinical care: a practical guide. *Diabet Med* 2019;36:803–812

121. Fegan-Bohm K, Minard CG, Anderson BJ, Butler AM, Titus C, Weissberg-Benchell J, et al. Diabetes distress and HbA1c in racially/ethnically and socioeconomically diverse youth with type 1 diabetes. Pediatr Diabetes. 2020;21(7):1362-9

122. Hilliard ME, Harris MA, Weissberg-Benchell J. Diabetes resilience: a model of risk and protection in type 1 diabetes. *Curr Diab Rep* 2012;12:739–748

123. Weissberg-Benchell J, Shapiro JB, Bryant FB, Hood KK. Supporting Teen Problem-Solving (STEPS) 3 year outcomes: preventing diabetes-specific emotional distress and depressive symptoms in adolescents with type 1 diabetes. *J Consult Clin Psychol* 2020;88:1019–1031

124. Gillham JE, Hamilton J, Freres DR, et al. Preventing depression among early adolescents in the primary care setting: a randomized controlled study of the Penn Resiliency Program. *J Abnorm Child Psychol* 2006;34:203–219

125 Fuller-Thomson E, Sawyer JL. Lifetime prevalence of suicidal ideation in a representative sample of Canadians with type 1 diabetes. *Diabetes Res Clin Pract* 2009;83:e9–e11

126. Butwicka A, Frisen L, Almqvist C, et al. Risks of psychiatric disorders and suicide attempts in children and adolescents with type 1 diabetes: a population-based cohort study. *Diabetes Care* 2015;38:453–459

127. Majidi S, O'Donnell HK, Stanek K, Youngkin E, Gomer T, Driscoll KA. Suicide risk assessment in youth and young adults with type 1 diabetes. *Diabetes Care.* 2020 Feb;43(2):343-348. doi: 10.2337/dc19-0831. Epub 2019 Dec 10. PMID: 31822488; PMCID: PMC6971783.

128. Pelkonen M, Marttunen M. Child and adolescent suicide: epidemiology, risk factors, and approaches to prevention. *Paediatr Drugs* 2003;5:243–265

129. Joiner TE. *Why People Die by Suicide.* Cambridge, MA, Harvard University Press, 2005

130. Van Orden KA, Witte TK, Cukrowicz KC, et al. The interpersonal theory of suicide. *Psychol Rev* 2010;117:575–600

131. Chu C, Klein KM, Buchman-Schmitt JM, et al. Routinized assessment of suicide risk in clinical practice: an empirically informed update. *J Clin Psychol* 2015;71:1186–1200

132. Gould MS, Marrocco FA, Kleinman M, et al. Evaluating iatrogenic risk of youth suicide screening programs: a randomized controlled trial. *JAMA* 2005;293:1635–1643

133. Dazzi T, Gribble R, Wessely S, Fear NT. Does asking about suicide and related behaviours induce suicidal ideation? What is the evidence? *Psychol Med* 2014;44:3361–3363

134. Gallagher ML, Miller AB. Suicidal thoughts and behavior in children and adolescents: an ecological model of resilience. *Adolesc Res Rev* 2018;3:123–154

135. Shahram SZ, Smith ML, Ben-David S, et al. Promoting "zest for life": a systematic literature review of resiliency factors to prevent youth suicide. *J Res Adolesc* 2021;31:4–24

136. Johansen NJ, Christensen MB. A systematic review on insulin overdose cases: clinical course, complications and treatment options. *Basic Clin Pharmacol Toxicol* 2018;122:650–659

137. Stanley B, Brown GK. Safety planning intervention: a brief intervention to mitigate suicide risk. *Cogn Behav Pract* 2012;19:256–264

138. Kroll J. Use of no-suicide contracts by psychiatrists in Minnesota. *Am J Psychiatry* 2000;157:1684–1686

139. Edwards SJ, Sachmann MD. No-suicide contracts, no-suicide agreements, and no-suicide assurances: a study of their nature, utilization, perceived effectiveness, and potential to cause harm. *Crisis* 2010;31:290–302

140. Rudd MD, Mandrusiak M, Joiner TE, Jr. The case against no-suicide contracts: the commitment to treatment statement as a practice alternative. *J Clin Psychol* 2006;62:243–251

141. Garvey KA, Penn JV, Campbell AL, et al. Contracting for safety with patients: clinical practice and forensic implications. *J Am Acad Psychiatry Law* 2009;37:363–370

142. Di Battista MA, Hart TA, Greco L, Gloizer J. Type 1 diabetes among adolescents: reduced diabetes self-care caused by social fear and fear of hypoglycemia. *Diabetes Educ* 2009;35:465–475

143. King KM, King PJ, Nayar R, Wilkes S. Perceptions of Adolescent patients of the "lived experience" of type 1 diabetes. *Diabetes Spectr* 2017;30:23–35

144. Main A, Wiebe DJ, Van Bogart K, et al. Secrecy from parents and type 1 diabetes management in late adolescence. *J Pediatr Psychol* 2015;40:1075–1084

145. Cox DJ, Irvine A, Gonder-Frederick L, et al. Fear of hypoglycemia: quantification, validation, and utilization. *Diabetes Care* 1987;10:617–621

146. Vallis M, Jones A, Pouwer F. Managing hypoglycemia in diabetes may be more fear management than glucose management: a practical guide for diabetes care providers. *Curr Diabetes Rev* 2014;10:364–370

147. Driscoll KA, Raymond J, Naranjo D, Patton SR. Fear of hypoglycemia in children and adolescents and their parents with type 1 diabetes. *Curr Diab Rep.* 2016 Aug;16(8):77. doi: 10.1007/s11892-016-0762-2. PMID: 27370530; PMCID: PMC5371512.

148. Gonder-Frederick LA, Fisher CD, Ritterband LM, et al. Predictors of fear of hypoglycemia in adolescents with type 1 diabetes and their parents. *Pediatr Diabetes.* 2006 Aug;7(4):215-22. doi: 10.1111/j.1399-5448.2006.00182.x. PMID: 16911009.

149. Shepard JA, Vajda K, Nyer M, Clarke W, Gonder-Frederick L. Understanding the construct of fear of hypoglycemia in pediatric type 1 diabetes. *J Pediatr Psychol.* 2014 Nov-Dec;39(10):1115-25. doi: 10.1093/jpepsy/jsu068. Epub 2014 Sep 11. PMID: 25214644; PMCID: PMC4201766.

150. O'Donnell HK, Bennett Johnson S, Sileo D, Majidi S, Gonder-Frederick L, Driscoll KA. Psychometric properties of the hypoglycemia fear survey in a clinical sample of adolescents with type 1 diabetes and their caregivers. *J Pediatr Psychol.* 2022 Feb 14;47(2):195-205. doi: 10.1093/jpepsy/jsab093. PMID: 34718681; PMCID: PMC8841982.

151. O'Donnell HK, Berget C, Wooldridge JS, Driscoll KA. Graduated exposure to treat fear of hypoglycemia in a young adult with type 1 diabetes: a case study. *Pediatr Diabetes* 2019;20:113–118

152. O'Donnell HK, Vigers T, Johnson SB, et al. Bring blood glucose down! An intervention to reduce fear of hypoglycemia in caregivers of adolescents with type 1 diabetes: Study design and participant characteristics. *Contemp Clin Trials.* 2022 Jul;118:106792. doi: 10.1016/j.cct.2022.106792. Epub 2022 May 16. PMID: 35589025.

153. Patton SR, McConville A, Marker AM, Monzon AD, Driscoll KA, Clements MA. Reducing emotional distress for childhood hypoglycemia in parents (REDCHiP): protocol for a randomized clinical trial to test a video-based telehealth intervention. *JMIR Res Protoc.* 2020 Aug 18;9(8):e17877. doi: 10.2196/17877. PMID: 32808936; PMCID: PMC7463405.

154. Cox DJ, Gonder-Frederick L, Polonsky W, et al. Blood glucose awareness training (BGAT-2): long-term benefits. *Diabetes Care* 2001;24:637–642

155. McMurtry CM, Pillai Riddell R, Taddio A, et al. Far from "just a poke": common painful needle procedures and the development of needle fear. *Clin J Pain* 2015;31:S3–S11

156. McLenon J, Rogers MAM. The fear of needles: a systematic review and meta-analysis. *J Adv Nurs* 2019;75:30–42

157. Duncanson E, Le Leu RK, Shanahan L, Macauley L, et al. The prevalence and evidence-based management of needle fear in adults with chronic disease: A scoping review. *PLoS One.* 2021 Jun 10;16(6):e0253048. doi: 10.1371/journal.pone.0253048. PMID: 34111207; PMCID: PMC8192004.

158. Howe CJ, Ratcliffe SJ, Tuttle A, et al. Needle anxiety in children with type 1 diabetes and their mothers. *MCN Am J Matern Child Nurs* 2011;36:25–31

159. Cemeroglu AP, Can A, Davis AT, et al. Fear of needles in children with type 1 diabetes mellitus on multiple daily injections and continuous subcutaneous insulin infusion. *Endocr Pract* 2015;21:46–53

160. McMurtry CM, Taddio A, Noel M, et al. Exposure-based interventions for the management of individuals with high levels of needle fear across the lifespan: a clinical practice guideline and call for further research. *Cogn Behav Ther* 2016;45:217–235

161. Zambanini A, Feher MD. Needle phobia in type 1 diabetes mellitus. *Diabet Med*. 1997 Apr;14(4):321-323.

162. Tran ST, Salamon KS, Hainsworth KR, et al. Pain reports in children and adolescents with type 1 diabetes mellitus. *J Child Health Care* 2015;19:43–52

163. Chambers CT, Taddio A, Uman LS, McMurtry CM. Psychological interventions for reducing pain and distress during routine childhood immunizations: a systematic review. *Clin Ther* 2009; 31(Suppl. 2):S77–S103

164. McMurtry CM, Chambers CT, McGrath PJ, Asp E. When "don't worry" communicates fear: children's perceptions of parental reassurance and distraction during a painful medical procedure. *Pain* 2010;150:52–58

165. Canbulat Sahiner N, Turkmen AS, Acikgoz A, et al. Effectiveness of two different methods for pain reduction during insulin injection in children with type 1 diabetes: Buzzy and ShotBlocker. *Worldviews Evid Based Nurs* 2018;15:464–470

166. Melzack R, Wall PD. Pain mechanisms: a new theory. *Science* 1965;150:971–979

167. Williams SE, Zahka NE. *Treating Somatic Symptoms in Children and Adolescents.* New York, Guilford Press, 2017

168. Reutrakul S, Thakkinstian A, Anothaisintawee T, et al. Sleep characteristics in type 1 diabetes and associations with glycemic control: systematic review and meta-analysis. *Sleep Med* 2016;23: 26–45

169. Monzon AD, Marker AM, Noser AE, et al. Associations between objective sleep behaviors and blood glucose variability in young children with type 1 diabetes. *Ann Behav Med* 2021;55:144–154

170. National Sleep Foundation. *Summary of Findings: 2006 Sleep In America Poll.* Washington, DC, National Sleep Foundation, 2006

171. Larcher S, Gauchez AS, Lablanche S, et al. Impact of sleep behavior on glycemic control in type 1 diabetes: the role of social jetlag. *Eur J Endocrinol* 2016;175:411–419

172. Roenneberg T, Kuehnle T, Pramstaller PP, et al. A marker for the end of adolescence. *Curr Biol* 2004;14:R1038–R1039

173. Wittmann M, Dinich J, Merrow M, Roenneberg T. Social jetlag: misalignment of biological and social time. *Chronobiol Int* 2006;23:497–509

174. von Schnurbein J, Boettcher C, Brandt S, et al. Sleep and glycemic control in adolescents with type 1 diabetes. *Pediatr Diabetes* 2018;19:143–149

175. Palmer CA, Oosterhoff B, Bower JL, et al. Associations among adolescent sleep problems, emotion regulation, and affective disorders: findings from a nationally representative sample. *J Psychiatr Res* 2018;96:1–8

176. Perfect MM, Patel PG, Scott RE, et al. Sleep, glucose, and daytime functioning in youth with type 1 diabetes. *Sleep* 2012;35:81–88

177. McDonough RJ, Clements MA, DeLurgio SA, Patton SR. Sleep duration and its impact on adherence in adolescents with type 1 diabetes mellitus. *Pediatr Diabetes* 2017;18:262–270

178. Sharifi A, De Bock MI, Jayawardene D, et al. Glycemia, treatment satisfaction, cognition, and sleep quality in adults and adolescents with type 1 diabetes when using a closed-loop system overnight versus sensor-augmented pump with low-glucose suspend function: a randomized crossover study. *Diabetes Technol Ther* 2016;18:772–783

179. Van Name MA, Hilliard ME, Boyle CT, et al. Nighttime is the worst time: parental fear of hypoglycemia in young children with type 1 diabetes. *Pediatr Diabetes* 2018;19:114–120

180. Deavin A, Greasley P, Dixon C. Children's perspectives on living with a sibling with a chronic illness. *Pediatrics* 2018;142:e20174151

181. Cao VT, Anderson BJ, Eshtehardi SS, et al. "We are a family with diabetes": parent perspectives on siblings of youth with type 1 diabetes. Fam Syst Health 2021;39:306–315

182. Herrman JW. Siblings' perceptions of the costs and rewards of diabetes and its treatment. *J Pediatr Nurs* 2010;25:428–437

183. Dougherty JP. The experience of siblings of children with type 1 diabetes. *Pediatr Nurs* 2015;41: 279–282, 305

184. Havill N, Fleming LK, Knafl K. Well siblings of children with chronic illness: A synthesis research study. *Res Nurs Health.* 2019 Oct;42(5):334-348. doi: 10.1002/nur.21978. Epub 2019 Aug 16. PMID: 31418465.

185. O'Brien I, Duffy A, Nicholl H. Impact of childhood chronic illnesses on siblings: a literature review. *Br J Nurs.* 2009 Dec 10-2010 Jan 13;18(22):1358, 1360-5. doi: 10.12968/bjon.2009.18.22.45562. PMID: 20081690.

CPSIA information can be obtained
at www.ICGtesting.com
Printed in the USA
JSHW050744270723
45478JS00001B/1

9 781580 408189